BEYOND THE CURE

BEYOND THE CURE

The Untold Stories of Antibiotics and How to Protect Yourself

Foreword by Brad Spellberg, MD, FIDSA

Henry Anyimadu, MD, FACP, FIDSA, AAHIVS

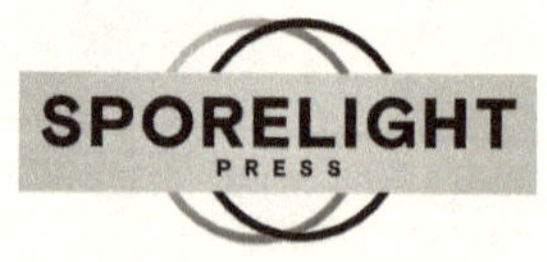

SPORELIGHT PRESS

Praise for Beyond the Cure

"A must-read for anyone who will ever need healthcare. "
—Paul Anthony, MD
System Director for Colleague Health Services,
Hartford HealthCare.

"Every day in healthcare, antibiotics are among the most common decisions we make and among the least examined for long-term harm. Beyond the Cure brings hidden risks to light through stories that speak to clinicians, patients, and families alike. It is exactly the kind of work we need if we are serious about building a culture of safety, stewardship, and trust. "
—Ajay Kumar, MD, MBA
Executive Vice President,
Chief Clinical Officer,
Hartford HealthCare

"A unique, masterfully crafted guide that helps readers protect themselves from the hidden pitfalls of antibiotics. Each chapter opens with a vivid story that grounds the science in real life and keeps you turning the pages. "
—Ophelia Chapman, DBA, MBA, MLIS
Associate Librarian,
University of North Carolina,
Wilmington

"Dr. Anyimadu has unlocked the true view on the yin and the yang that accompanies antibiotics, showing through compelling stories the life-saving properties of this miracle cure as well as the downside of performing such miracles. He has an incredible grasp on the subject matter that is a must-read for all."
—Ulysses Wu, MD
Chief Antibiotic Steward,
System Director for Infectious Diseases,
Hartford HealthCare

"Beyond the Cure reveals the delicate balance between the life-saving power of antibiotics and the sometimes life-altering harms they can cause, even with the best-intended care. Through vivid patient stories, it turns stewardship principles into clear, practical guidance for clinicians and the public."
—Kevin D. Dieckhaus, MD, FIDSA
Professor of Medicine,
Chief, Division of Infectious Diseases,
Director of Global Health & International Studies,
UConn Health

"Well written and compelling, Beyond the Cure is a practical, case-based guide to the infectious disease dilemmas clinicians face every day and the antibiotic decisions that shape patient outcomes. Dr. Anyimadu brings decades of experience to a poignant, enlightening read that is essential for anyone concerned about their health and the future of healthcare."
—Lisa M. Chirch, MD, FIDSA
Professor of Medicine; Fellowship Director,
Division of Infectious Diseases University of Connecticut,
School of Medicine

"Beyond the Cure is a timely and essential work that confronts the hidden costs of antibiotic use with honesty, compassion, and clinical rigor. Through powerful stories and clear evidence, Dr. Anyimadu reminds us that good medicine is not just about treating disease, but about humility, stewardship, and respect for the human body. This book should be required reading for clinicians and deeply empowering for patients. "
—**Mohammed Shams, MD, MBA**
Regional Chair of Medicine

"Through vivid, compelling storytelling, Beyond the Cure shines a spotlight on one of the most transformative medical and public health breakthroughs of the modern era, antibiotics. The book explores their extraordinary life-saving power while thoughtfully confronting the challenges that accompany their use, including medication risks and the growing threat of antibiotic resistance. By seamlessly weaving clear scientific insight with real-world stories, Dr. Anyimadu demystifies a complex topic, making it both engaging and accessible for clinicians and general readers alike. "
—**David Banach MD, MPH**
Hospital Epidemiologist,
Professor of Medicine,
University of Connecticut,
School of Medicine

"Our communities depend on us not only to treat infections today, but to preserve the power of antibiotics for tomorrow. Beyond the Cure empowers clinicians and patients with shared language to do both. This is exactly the kind of honest, story-driven work we need to change culture. Beyond the Cure shows how safer, personalized antibiotic use can protect individual patients and strengthen trust in our entire health system. "

—Gina Coleman, MBA, MPH, FACHE
President,
Central Region,
Hartford HealthCare

Dedication

To the Author of life and healing, to God be the glory. Every page of this book, like every breath, is a gift of grace.
To my wife, Nana Adwoa, my steady anchor and closest friend. Your faith keeps my compass true.
To my children, Afia, Gabriel, and Joel, my daily joy and most cherished legacy.
And to the one whose love still surrounds us.
This book is for all of you who have walked with me, not only beyond the cure, but toward what truly matters.

Contents

Foreword

Antibiotics are the most lifesaving interventions in the millennia-long history of medicine.

Nothing else has ever come close to their power to save lives. Before antibiotics became available in the 1930s, common diseases killed with regularity and impunity, and people routinely died young from such infections. Physicians had little to offer beyond placebos—or treatments that did more harm than good. With the arrival of antibiotics, suddenly, after thousands of years of placebos and harmful nonsense, doctors acquired the power to reliably cure deadly diseases. Lifespans began to be significantly prolonged. Medicine was off and running.

But there is a dark side to this nearly effortless power that antibiotics give to doctors to cure ailments. And it is this dark side that Dr. Anyimadu addresses so effectively in Beyond the Cure. Antibiotics are so powerful and so widely available that they are just too easy to prescribe and take. The result? Doctors and patients abuse these drugs with alarming regularity. We use them to treat our own anxiety about illness, even when the illness is not caused by bacteria, and the antibiotic cannot possibly help. Antibiotics make us feel safe. They make us feel like we are doing something, even when we are not.

Unfortunately, every single use of an antibiotic increases the risk of the emergence of resistance to the antibiotic. The more we use them, the less effective they become. If we are truly treating dangerous bacterial infections, the risk of triggering resistance is worth taking because we are curing an illness that could kill the patient. But when we give antibiotics to patients who don't need them, we assume the same risk of increasing antibiotic resistance without any offsetting benefit. In these cases, we accelerate antibiotic resistance and erode the effectiveness of these drugs to cure people who truly need them. Widespread unnecessary use threatens to send us back to the pre-antibiotic era, losing the miraculous power of antibiotics to cure disease.

And as Dr. Anyimadu explains in Beyond the Cure, rising antibiotic resistance is not the only risk. Because, along with their incredible power to cure disease, antibiotics can also cause dangerous side effects. Some can injure the kidneys. Some can injure the liver. Some can cause dangerous heart arrhythmias. Some cause dangerous allergic reactions. And all wipe out the good bacteria that normally live in our bodies, predisposing the patient to dangerous super-infections caused by other pathogens. Thus, the belief that antibiotics are only good and never cause harm is not only naïve—it is wrong.

Dr. Anyimadu has put together an educational manual to teach people about the harms of antibiotics and to help them balance their faith in their curative power. This is a hard conversation to have. And it addresses behaviors that are very hard to change. But we must change them if we wish to continue to have these drugs available to cure real diseases in the future. Beyond the Cure is an important contribution to this effort.

Brad Spellberg, MD
Chief Medical Officer
Los Angeles General Medical Center

Author of:
1. *Rising Plague: The Global Threat from Deadly Bacteria and Our Dwindling Arsenal to Fight Them*
2. *Broken, Bankrupt, and Dying: How to Solve the Great American Healthcare Rip-Off*

Preface

On a night when New York felt a world away from home, I sat on the edge of a narrow dorm bed with a phone pressed to my ear, listening as my mother tried to be brave. Her voice was thin. A new medicine had set her hands on fire. Her feet blistered. Sleep was a stranger. The plan had been simple: start a powerful drug now, fine-tune the diagnosis later. When the pathology finally arrived, the truth cut both ways. The disease was milder than feared. My mother's suffering had been needless.

I hung up and stared at the ceiling for a long time. As a son, I felt grief and a kind of quiet fury. As a young physician, I felt something else settle in that would not leave. We do not always know the whole story when we reach for a prescription. We act to protect, yet our actions can wound. In the clinic, certainty is a luxury. Pills are easy to start and hard to question. Collateral damage is real and too often invisible.

Antibiotics sit at the very center of this tension. They have turned death sentences into detours and saved more lives than any single class of drugs in history. They have also been used when they were not needed, used longer than necessary, and used without regard for the quiet ecosystems inside us that keep us well. Up to half of today's antibiotic prescriptions are unnecessary or misdirected. That is not a small footnote in modern medicine. That is a fault line.

This book begins at that fault line. *Beyond the Cure* invites you into rooms where decisions are made with incomplete maps and real consequences. You will meet patients who did everything right and were harmed anyway.

You will stand beside clinicians who balance one person's relief against another person's future.

You will see how a routine pill can unsettle a liver or redraw a gut's landscape. You will also see how small, steady changes in how we diagnose, prescribe, and prevent can spare suffering and keep our best medicines strong.

If you are a patient, this book offers language and questions that make your care safer. If you are a parent, it offers a way to weigh fear against facts. If you are a clinician, it offers a mirror and practical tools for the days when habit wants the pen more than evidence does. If you are a student of any kind, it offers a way to see medicine not as magic but as disciplined compassion.

I wrote these pages to tell untold stories, but also to point toward a better way. Rapid diagnostics can replace guessing. Shorter courses can work as well as long ones. Prevention can do what no drug ever will. New science, including machine learning, can help us choose precisely and stop on time.

I invite you to join me as we explore these untold stories. Understanding the whole truth about antibiotics doesn't diminish their power; it deepens our appreciation, sharpens our judgment, and guides us toward safer and wiser use. If by the end you wash your hands more intentionally, ask a better question at a clinic visit, stop a prescription two days earlier when the evidence says it is enough, or choose to prevent an infection rather than chase it later, then the work of this book will have mattered.

This is not the story I expected to tell. It is the one I needed to tell. I am grateful you are here.

Author's Note

Out of respect for the privacy of the individuals whose stories appear in this book, and in accordance with the Health Insurance Portability and Accountability Act (HIPAA), names, settings, and identifying details have been altered to protect confidentiality. Some clinical scenarios are composites, and often timelines have been condensed to protect confidentiality without changing clinical meaning.

The views, opinions, and interpretations in *Beyond the Cure: The Untold Stories of Antibiotics* are solely those of the author. They do not represent the policies, positions, or endorsements of Hartford HealthCare, the University of Connecticut, the Infectious Diseases Society of America, or any affiliated institutions. Any endorsements included are from individuals in their personal capacity, not on behalf of their institutions. This book is intended for educational and reflective purposes. It is not medical advice, does not replace consultation with a qualified clinician, and does not establish a physician–patient relationship.

Henry Anyimadu, MD, FACP, FIDSA, AAHIVS
Chief of Infectious Diseases,
Hartford HealthCare,
Central Region

Chapter 1

Poor Liver

The Son of Accra

On Harmattan mornings in Accra, Ghana, when the wind blows dust soft as flour across the city, Kwame Adu used to step out into the light with a cloth over his shoulder and a list in his head. He grew up between the bustle of Kaneshie Market and the sea-breeze evenings of Jamestown, where the lighthouse blinks its patient eye over wooden canoes.

As a boy, he ran errands on tro-tro minibuses, cedi notes folded neatly in his palm. As a man, he sold electrical parts near Makola, ate waakye wrapped in banana leaves, and

never missed a Hearts of Oak match if he could help it. He was careful in the Ghanaian way, meticulous with money, generous with neighbors, proud of a body that had served him without complaint.

When Kwame left for America, he carried two suitcases and three promises: work hard, send money home, stay healthy. For nearly a decade, he kept all three. Mornings started before sunrise with a thermos of Milo, nights ended late, boots by the door, and phone calls to Accra crackling through five time zones. At sixty, his primary care doctor called him "remarkably fit." Strong heart. Clear lungs. The stamina of a man half his age.

So when a routine immigration physical included a test for tuberculosis (TB), standard for many who have lived where TB is common, Kwame treated it like any other form to fill. He had no cough, no fever, no night sweats. He felt fine. The result came back: latent TB infection—no active disease, no risk to others, but a small chance the sleeping bacteria could wake someday.

"It is common," his doctor said kindly. "We see this a lot in people who grew up in West Africa. The safest path is preventive treatment. One pill a day for a few months. "

Kwame nodded. In Accra, he had learned to act before trouble arrived, repair a cracked step before the rains, service the generator before the lights go out. He agreed to start isoniazid (also known as isonicotinic acid hydrazide, or INH). His liver tests were normal. The plan felt simple, a pill for peace of mind.

But under Kwame's right ribs, the quiet sentinel that filters, stores, and steadies (the liver) was about to protest.

Most of us rarely think about the liver. It does not thump like the heart or flash like the brain. Yet it is the city's busiest roundabout, with more than five hundred tasks circling through at once, turning food into fuel, corralling toxins, managing hormones, and helping blood clot. It is sturdy and forgiving, and it can regenerate even after serious injury. Precisely because it seldom complains, we miss its whispers until they become a shout.

The first hints are easy to ignore: a heaviness after meals, a quiet fatigue, a touch of nausea you might blame on a late dinner or a long week. Kwame waved those away. He had pushed through worse back home when inventory arrived late, or the lights flickered off mid-sale.

Then one morning, weeks into treatment, he leaned toward the bathroom mirror and stopped. The whites of his eyes were no longer white; they had turned yellow. His urine had turned dark, tea colored. The whispers were shouting.

In the emergency department, the triage nurse saw the yellow and moved quickly. Bloodwork told the story: liver enzymes soaring, bilirubin rising, the chemistry of a sentinel under siege. INH, a medicine that protects thousands, has a rare but real capacity to injure the liver, especially in older adults. They stopped the drug at once. They watched. They hoped.

By evening, his belly was swelling with fluid. Toxins that the liver usually clears began to cloud his thinking. Words slipped from his grasp like fish through a torn net. The ICU team spoke softly about acute liver failure, about transplantation, about time—a resource they were running out of.

Kwame's heart faltered. A code was called. For twenty-four long minutes, a roomful of strangers refused to let go, and his pulse returned. A fragile victory. But his kidneys had joined the protest. Dialysis was started (a process of cleaning out toxins from the body). Machines hummed. Family gathered, holding hands as they had at church in Osu, Accra, and at funerals under white tents. Near dawn, with monitors tracing thin lines and prayers rising in two countries at once, Kwame Adu's heart grew quiet for the last time.

I was a young trainee on that service. I stood at the edge of the room, learning the choreography of crisis and the limits of our certainty. Later, as I wrote the note no family ever wants to read, a question lodged itself in my mind and has never left:

Did Kwame need the pill that ended his life?

Latent TB is common. Nearly a quarter of the world carries it silently. Most will never fall ill. Preventive therapy saves lives in people at higher risk; those with recent exposure, weak immune systems, or other conditions that tilt the odds toward reactivation. But Kwame was sixty, healthy, and years removed from likely exposure. He deserved a conversation that weighed his small personal risk of active TB against his age-related risk of drug-induced liver injury, and that offered alternatives with lower liver toxicity and shorter courses. He also deserved the most explicit warning we can give: If you are nauseous, your appetite vanishes, your urine darkens, your eyes yellow, stop the medicine and call today, not tomorrow. Guidelines are maps, not marching orders. They point the way, and the person in front of us decides the route.

In Accra, they say, "When you carry someone, you feel their weight." Medicine must do the same. We must feel the weight of the individual—their age, history, and hopes—before we set a pill on their tongue.

Kwame's story is not an indictment of prevention. It is a plea for precision and humility. Every powerful drug is a double-edged blade. We honor its force by using it right-sized and right-timed, by listening for the liver's whisper before it becomes a scream, by making room for second opinions and shared decisions, and by choosing the safest effective option whenever there is a choice.

This book begins here, at a bedside where good intentions met a hidden cost, because Beyond the Cure is about everything that happens before and after an antibiotic is prescribed. It is about stories and habits that prevent illness, and the questions that keep us safe when medicine is needed. It is about remembering that behind every guideline is a human life, and behind every liver enzyme is a father, a friend, a full name:

Kwame Adu, son of Accra, who taught us, at a cost we will never forget, that the liver is loyal but not limitless.

The Chemistry

In the 1960s, chemists at the Beecham Group were quietly refining penicillin's blueprint when they arrived at amoxicillin, a semisynthetic cousin built for reliability. It absorbed well by mouth, reached tissues quickly, was effective against many pathogens, and was gentle enough for broad use. When it reached pharmacies in 1972, general practitioners and hospital teams alike embraced it. Sore throats, ear infections, skin and urinary infections that once lingered now cleared with predictable speed. For a time, it felt as if a smarter penicillin had finally arrived.

Bacteria, however, study us as intently as we study them. In clinic after clinic, strains of staphylococci and gram-negative rods began producing beta-lactamase, an enzyme that snapped open amoxicillin's ring and left it useless. The drug still worked where that enzyme was absent, but the cracks were visible.

Beecham researchers returned to the lab bench and found an unexpected ally in a soil microbe, Streptomyces clavuligerus. From it, they isolated clavulanic acid, a small molecule that binds and disables many beta-lactamases. The idea was elegant. Pair the time-tested antibiotic with a guardian that neutralizes the enzyme long enough for the antibiotic to do its work.

That pairing became amoxicillin–clavulanate, first marketed in the United Kingdom in 1981 under the name Augmentin and approved by the U.S. Food and Drug Administration in 1984. In practice, the combination restored activity against many common beta-lactamase producers, turning clinical dead ends back into straightforward cures. It did not solve every problem, and it was never meant to be used for everything. Still, it marked a turning point: an early proof that judicious chemistry could outmaneuver resistance, at least for a while, by protecting an old drug with a precisely chosen partner.

The chemistry came first: amoxicillin paired with clavulanate, an elegant team that rescued a good drug from the enzymes that had begun to blunt it. By the early 1980s, Augmentin sat in doctors' bags from London to Long Island, restoring cures where simple penicillins had started to fail.

It was never meant to be a hammer for every nail. It was a sharper tool for jobs that needed it. Sharp tools, used often enough, can still cut the wrong way.

Jim, the yellow New Yorker

On a brisk October morning in Manhattan, Jim Marshall hustled down Eighth Avenue with a paper cup of coffee warming his hands. He was forty-eight, a project manager who split his weekdays between Midtown meetings and late-night emails at a kitchen table overlooking a slice of West Side sky. New York had taught him to keep moving. He ran loops around the reservoir, squeezed onto uptown trains, and timed school drop-offs to the minute. When he caught a sinus infection, he refused to give in. His symptoms persisted for well over a week. His primary care doctor on the Upper West Side explained that viruses commonly cause sinusitis, but sometimes bacteria can cause it, too. Since his symptoms had persisted for well over a week, he wrote a familiar prescription: Augmentin. Jim hardly thought about it. His kids had taken it for ear infections. A coworker swore it cleared her chest cold. He picked up the blister pack at the corner pharmacy, grabbed a deli sandwich, and swallowed the first pill between calls.

The first couple of days felt reassuring. The pressure eased. Sleep returned. He tolerated the usual annoyances—softer stools and a little fatigue—and by day seven he was planning a Sunday run in Central Park to make up for lost miles. He finished the ten-day course, left the bottle on his kitchen counter, and continued with life.

A week later, Jim woke up to find the mirror reflecting a stranger's face. The whites of his eyes had a telltale yellow tint. His skin, normally ruddy from outdoor work, looked like faded parchment. At first, he thought it was a trick of the light. But by midmorning, nausea and an odd itchiness under his skin forced him to call in sick. His urine darkened to the color of cola. Jim's wife insisted they go to the ER, and, for once, he didn't argue.

At the hospital, chaos replaced routine. Nurses drew vial after vial of blood. Doctors frowned at computer screens showing wildly abnormal liver tests. His liver enzymes and bilirubin levels were twenty times higher than normal. One doctor murmured about hepatitis, the kind caused by viruses.

But every hepatitis test came back negative. As the day wore on, Jim's eyes turned a deeper yellow.

By evening, a senior physician, Dr. Patel, pulled up a chair at Jim's bedside. She spoke in a calm, steady voice that made the words no less shocking: "Jim, your liver is in trouble. We think the antibiotic you took—the Augmentin—triggered a rare reaction. In short, the medicine that was supposed to help you is now hurting your liver." Jim was floored. My antibiotic did this? He had trusted those pills implicitly. Antibiotics were benign, weren't they? They cured infections; they didn't put you in a hospital bed, jaundiced and weak. As he grappled with this reversal of expectations, Dr. Patel explained that he was suffering from what doctors call drug-induced liver injury, or DILI. It's a rare side effect, she said gently, but not unheard of with Augmentin. His liver had become inflamed and was unable to do its job of filtering toxins.

The yellow hue overtaking his body was caused by bilirubin, a waste product his sick liver could no longer clear. Jim was full of fear and anger. He pictured his kids at home, wondering where Dad was, and his mind kept circling back to the empty bottle of antibiotics on the kitchen counter. How could a simple course of antibiotics, the same kind thousands of people take every day for sinus or ear infections, land him here, fighting for his life? Over the next two days, Jim's condition teetered on the edge. His liver was in acute rebellion. Every eight hours, the medical team checked his lab results, hoping to see a downward trend in those liver enzymes and bilirubin.

They spoke in hushed tones about the possibility of a liver transplant if things didn't turn around, a prospect that terrified Jim. Each passing hour felt like a pendulum swing between disaster and relief.

Late on the third day, a slight dip in those enzyme levels sparked cautious optimism. Jim's liver had stopped worsening; it might just heal itself if given time. Lying in his hospital bed, Jim kept asking himself and anyone who'd listen: How did this happen? *How could a medication as common as Augmentin nearly cause my liver to fail?* To answer that, Dr. Patel went back to basics.

She described how the liver is the body's chemical factory, processing almost everything we eat or drink, and every pill we swallow. "Think of it as the body's filter and pharmacy in one," she said. When Jim took Augmentin, his liver's job was to break down the antibiotic into forms that could be excreted safely. But in rare instances, those breakdown products aren't so harmless. In Jim's case, his immune system likely misidentified some fragment of the drug as dangerous and launched an attack, not just on the drug but on his own liver cells. It was a microscopic case of friendly fire.

This kind of reaction, Dr. Patel explained, is idiosyncratic, a big word for a simple idea: unpredictable and personal. If you give a thousand people the same antibiotic, 999 will likely process it just fine. But one unlucky person might have their liver ambushed by their body's own defenses. It's not about overdose or misuse; Jim followed the directions to the letter. In fact, doctors contrast it with something like a Tylenol overdose, which is a predictable liver injury where too much of the drug will damage anyone's liver. Jim's case was the opposite, a bolt from the blue. Rare, unpredictable, but very real.

As Jim slowly recovered, he learned that his story, while uncommon, was not a bizarre one-in-a-million fluke. In the world of medicine, Augmentin had long been on the radar of liver specialists. It turns out Augmentin is one of the leading causes of antibiotic-related liver injury worldwide. One might expect exotic, experimental drugs to top that list, but here was an everyday antibiotic taking that dubious honor. In fact, by some estimates, Augmentin has become the single most common cause of acute drug-induced liver injury in the United States and Europe. The reason is not because it's exceptionally toxic to everyone; millions take it safely, but because it's prescribed so widely, those rare one-in-a-few-thousand chances add up to a lot of people.

To put it in perspective, doctors write antibiotic prescriptions in huge numbers, tens of millions each year in the United States alone. Most people pop the pills, maybe get a bit of an upset stomach, and that's the end of it. But if even a fraction of a percent experience severe liver injury, that's still hundreds or thousands of patients facing what Jim did.

According to one large study, the mortality rate for patients who suffer antibiotic-triggered liver failure can be as high as 14%, a sobering statistic that underscores how high the stakes are when things go wrong. Jim was fortunate; he recovered without needing a transplant. Many others aren't so lucky. In 2024, a team of researchers decided to quantify just how big this problem is.

They combed through electronic health records of nearly eight million patients over two decades, looking for patterns. The results, published in JAMA Internal Medicine, were eye-opening. Out of hundreds of medications studied, many known to have potential liver side effects, antibiotics stood out prominently. In fact, six of the top seventeen drugs most likely to send someone to the hospital with acute liver injury were common antibiotics.

And, yes, Augmentin was one of them, confirming what liver specialists had long suspected. But it wasn't alone on that list: There were sulfa antibiotics like Bactrim, fluoroquinolones like ciprofloxacin and levofloxacin, and even a macrolide antibiotic similar to the popular Z-pack. These are medications millions of people have taken for a urinary tract infection, a respiratory infection, or even acne. It's not just Augmentin, Bactrim, or ciprofloxacin, either. History is dotted with examples of antibiotics that turned out to carry heavy risks for the liver.

Dr. Patel told Jim about a drug called trovafloxacin, a powerful antibiotic introduced in the late 1990s with great fanfare. Trovafloxacin, sold as Trovan, was meant to be a triumph against serious infections. But within a year of its release, reports started emerging of patients developing fulminant (sudden and severe) liver failure. Over 140 cases of serious liver damage were eventually attributed to Trovan, including more than a dozen acute liver failure deaths. It was a catastrophe. By 1999, Trovan was taken off the market for use in all but life-threatening situations. A miracle drug turned menace almost overnight. These stories left Jim with a paradox to wrestle with: Antibiotics can both heal and kill. After his recovery, Jim found a new perspective. He felt gratitude that antibiotics exist at all; without them, a simple sinus infection could turn deadly. But he also felt a healthy respect for the power of these drugs. He realized that "safe" doesn't mean risk-free.

Every medication is a balancing act between help and harm. To Jim, the harm to the liver was very concerning because we don't see or feel our liver most of the time; these injuries remain an unseen danger, quietly occurring in hospital wards and described in specialist journals. They are the untold stories behind the cures. After a week in the hospital and another month of recuperation at home, Jim's life gradually returned to normal. His skin cleared, and his strength returned. Within a month, he felt like himself again. But he wasn't quite the same person who had casually taken an antibiotic without a second thought. Before his discharge, Dr. Patel shared one final thought that stayed with him.

"Your liver should recover fully," she said. "Remember your gut. Antibiotics do not just hit the bug in your sinus. They ripple through the trillions of bacteria that live in you. That microbiome helps digest food, make vitamins, and keep other infections at bay. After a course like this, your gut can look like a forest after a fire. It grows back, but the mix can be different for a while. "

He tucked that away while focusing on healing, but the image would not leave. A forest after a fire. An unseen world changed by a week of pills.

Jim's story is not here to frighten anyone away from antibiotics. It is here to restore respect. Ask before you swallow the first dose. Do I really need this drug? What are the risks, even if they're rare? And how many days are enough? For clinicians, his chart is a nudge to watch for the one patient in a thousand whose eyes turn yellow, and to stop the medicine before the whisper becomes a shout. For all of us, his recovery opens the next door in this book.

Key ideas

- Some antibiotics can inflame the liver; early symptoms are subtle.
- Risk rises with alcohol use, preexisting liver disease, and polypharmacy.
- Lab monitoring and clear stop dates reduce harm.

Do this — Readers

- Keep a current medication list (including herbals and over-the-counter medications); share it at every visit.
- Ask: "Does this drug affect the liver? Do I need lab tests?"
- Avoid alcohol while on antibiotics unless your clinician says otherwise.
- Watch for dark urine, right upper abdominal pain, itching, or yellow eyes; call promptly.
- Confirm the stop date and set a phone reminder.

Do this — Clinicians

- Check baseline liver enzymes, medical history, medications, alcohol use; document stop dates.
- Prefer agents with safer hepatic profiles when options exist.
- Order targeted lab tests for at-risk patients; teach them the warning signs.
- Reconcile medications; avoid duplicate hepatotoxins.

Conversation starters

- "What's my liver risk with this antibiotic?"
- "When will we do lab tests?"

Chapter 2

Gut Feeling

Ms. Jay awoke in her hospital room with a cautious sense of relief. At seventy-six years old, she had just come through a successful hip replacement surgery. The hardest part, she thought, should be over. As a retired teacher and proud grandmother, she was eager to get back on her feet literally, so she could chase after her toddling grandson at the next family gathering. But in the days following her surgery, a gut feeling told her something wasn't right. It started as a dull ache in her abdomen, then grew into painful cramps and waves of nausea. Nurses noticed she wasn't her usual chatty self. By the third day, Ms. Jay was wracked with fever and urgently ill with terrible diarrhea that wouldn't stop. The staff hurried to isolate her in a single room, donning gowns and gloves as if entering a danger zone. Ms. Jay's relief turned to alarm. *What is happening to me?* she wondered, frightened and alone.

In a matter of hours, this feisty, independent woman became so weak she could barely shuffle to the bathroom. Embarrassment and fear weighed on her with every trip; it felt like her body was betraying her. The doctors initially suspected a common postoperative infection, maybe something she picked up during surgery. They ordered tests and started a broad-spectrum antibiotic to fight whatever was causing the fever. Ms. Jay dutifully swallowed the pills, trusting they would make her better. Instead, her symptoms worsened. Her diarrhea became explosive, and severe cramps doubled her over in pain.

Dehydration sapped her strength; her mouth felt dry as cotton, and she grew disoriented.

I survived surgery, only to be laid low by this? she thought in despair, clutching her aching belly.

Finally, a lab result came back that explained the nightmare. Ms. Jay had tested positive for *Clostridioides difficile*, a bacterium she had never heard of before. Commonly called *C. diff*, it was an infection likely triggered by the very antibiotics meant to protect her. The antibiotic she'd been given after surgery had wiped out many of the "good" bacteria in her gut, the friendly microbes that normally keep bad germs in check. In that void, *C. diff* had flourished like weeds in a garden cleared of plants. Now this aggressive bacteria was inflaming her colon and releasing toxins, causing intense pain and life-threatening diarrhea. Ms. Jay was stunned. She had gone to the hospital to fix a hip, and now a microscopic bug was threatening her life.

The doctors immediately stopped the broad-spectrum antibiotic that had unknowingly opened the door to infection. Instead, they started Ms. Jay on a specific antibiotic targeted for *C. diff*. It felt ironic to her—another antibiotic to treat a problem caused by antibiotics. She received oral vancomycin, and within a few days her fever dropped and the flow of diarrhea slowed. Weak and shaken, Ms. Jay was relieved to be improving, but the experience had traumatized her. *Will this really cure it? Will it come back?* she wondered. Each day, she felt a bit stronger and was eventually discharged from the hospital to continue recovering at home with her daughter's help.

For a couple of weeks, life slowly returned to normal. Ms. Jay managed to eat bland foods and stay hydrated. She even took short walks in her garden, grateful for simple pleasures like sunlight and fresh air after her harrowing ordeal. But that gratitude was short-lived. About a month after the hospital, her symptoms suddenly returned—the cramping, fever, and yes, the awful diarrhea. Ms. Jay's heart sank; it was déjà vu. Her doctor confirmed her fear: The *C. diff* infection was back. This pattern repeated itself again in the coming weeks. Each time, she would endure the indignity and pain of the infection, take her medicine, feel better for a while, and then get sick once more. Ms. Jay began to wonder if she would ever truly be well again. "Do you think I will ever be rid of this awful *C. diff*?" she asked her infectious disease specialist in a trembling voice during yet another clinic visit.

She wasn't just physically exhausted; the illness was wearing down her spirit.

Her doctor offered a gentle smile. He explained that *C. diff* recurrences are common, but there was hope. Each recurrence was not her fault; it was the nature of this stubborn infection. The *C. diff* bacteria produce hardy spores that can linger in the gut and the environment. Even after initial treatment wipes out active bacteria, dormant spores can survive and reignite the infection once the medication is stopped. Ms. Jay learned that it takes time, sometimes months, for the normal balance of gut bacteria to fully recover leaving her vulnerable during that period.

The specialist reassured her that, with patience, her gut's "good" flora would rebound and help keep *C. diff* at bay. In the meantime, they would be cautious with further antibiotics and focus on supportive care. He also emphasized strict hygiene at home to avoid spreading the germ to others. Ms. Jay's daughter diligently cleaned every surface with bleach-based products and made sure everyone washed their hands meticulously. They were determined to fight this unseen enemy and would not let it claim victory.

Slowly but surely, Ms. Jay's body fought back. Her doctors decided to try a new plan; vancomycin was given in a tapered and pulsed regimen over several weeks to ensure any lingering *C. diff* spores were eradicated. This time, the infection finally loosened its grip. Ms. Jay went week after week with no symptoms. Her strength began to return. One sunny afternoon, about four months after the nightmare began, she found herself back in her garden, pruning her beloved rose bushes. A wave of emotion came over her as she realized she felt *normal* again. Tears of relief welled up; she had her life back. Ms. Jay's journey through hell and back opened her eyes to an alarming truth: Something as routine as an antibiotic prescription had nearly killed her. It was a wake-up call that left her determined to share her story and prevent others from suffering the same fate.

As Ms. Jay slowly recovered, another story of antibiotics and unintended consequences was unfolding hundreds of miles away. Anna Carter was a thirty-two-year-old mother of two and a busy marketing professional in the prime of her life. Anna always thought of antibiotics as harmless magic pills—you take them for a nasty sinus infection or a persistent cough, and in a few days you're back to normal. She had never imagined that a simple course of pills could unleash a chain reaction that would throw her world into chaos.

It all started with a bad case of strep throat. Juggling work deadlines and her kids' schedules, Anna tried to power through the soreness and fever, but eventually conceded that she needed medicine. Her doctor prescribed a ten-day course of cephalexin (commonly known as Keflex) to wipe out the infection. At first, the drug worked as expected—her throat pain subsided, and she was back at the office within a week, boasting to colleagues about the "wonders of modern medicine." But about a month later, Anna began experiencing bizarre digestive issues. She had sudden bouts of cramping and had to run to the bathroom multiple times a day. Food seemed to race through her, and she joked to her husband that she must have caught a "24-hour stomach bug." When the symptoms persisted into the second and third day, Anna's joke turned into genuine worry.

Over the next week, life for Anna became a nightmare. She grew weaker each day, hardly able to eat. At night, she'd wake up drenched in sweat, then shiver with chills—a sign of fever. The bathroom was now her most frequented room. It was as if that "stomach bug" had made a permanent home in her gut. Her family watched in concern as outgoing, energetic Anna became a shell of herself. She lost weight; dark circles formed under her eyes. Still, ER doctors initially brushed it off as a viral gastroenteritis (a typical stomach flu). She was told to stay hydrated and ride it out. But Anna's intuition told her this was no ordinary bug. She felt something was terribly wrong inside, a deep gut instinct that this illness was different. Desperate for answers, she visited an urgent care clinic where, thankfully, one attentive physician took her symptoms seriously. They ran tests—blood work and a stool culture. Anna was sent home with a tentative diagnosis of possible *C. diff* infection, pending lab confirmation, and instructions to start oral vancomycin if the results came back positive.

When the phone rang the next morning, confirming *C. diff*, Anna felt a mix of weird relief and new fear. Relief, because finally she had a name for this torment. Fear, because a quick internet search told her that *Clostridioides difficile* was a notoriously nasty infection. She learned that *C. diff* often strikes people after antibiotic use, when beneficial gut bacteria are wiped out, and this opportunistic germ takes over.

It can cause anything from mild diarrhea to life-threatening colitis. Reading further, Anna's jaw dropped at the statistics: Hundreds of thousands of people get sick from it each year, and tens of thousands die.

"How on earth did I end up with this?" she murmured. She was a young, healthy woman who had simply taken antibiotics for a common infection. It was eye-opening—and terrifying—to realize that the cure she took for strep throat had opened the door to an even worse illness.

The next few weeks were some of the hardest of Anna's life. Vancomycin in hand, she battled the *C. diff* head-on.

The medication gradually helped calm the intestinal storm; the fevers eased, and her bowel movements started to normalize. But the treatment itself was no picnic. The pills left an unpleasant taste in her mouth and sometimes gave her headaches and nausea. She read the fine print of the drug information and winced at warnings of potential side effects. It seemed cruelly fitting: The remedy carried its own risks. Still, she persisted, clinging to the hope of a normal life on the other side of this ordeal.

Anna's two little children were kept at a careful distance while Mom recovered. She'd blow them kisses from her bed, aching not just in her gut but in her heart because she couldn't hug them for fear of spreading germs. Her husband became Mr. Mom overnight—cooking meals, cleaning the house with hospital-grade disinfectant, and helping Anna however he could. Emotionally, Anna felt wrung out. The illness isolated her at a time when she needed comfort the most. In quiet moments, her mind wandered to dark places: *What if I don't get better? What if it keeps coming back?* She had read about people suffering recurrent *C. diff* infections, some facing recurrence after recurrence, trapped in a cycle of sickness.

The thought of living in permanent fear of this lurking bacteria was overwhelming.

Sure enough, about two weeks after finishing her medication, Anna's symptoms roared back. It was like a cruel joke. One evening, she sat down to dinner, only to be struck with sharp abdominal pains halfway through the meal. Within hours, she was running to the bathroom again. *Not now, not again,* she thought, tears in her eyes. A test confirmed the *C. diff* was back for an encore. Her doctor explained that roughly one in five patients experience a recurrence after an initial infection, and some unlucky folks, especially younger, otherwise healthy individuals like her, were increasingly getting *C. diff* outside of hospital settings. This was no longer just a hospital-acquired infection affecting elderly patients; it could strike anyone, anywhere, given the right conditions. Anna refused to surrender to despair. With her doctor's guidance, she dove into a new treatment plan to vanquish the resilient intruder.

This time, they tried another treatment called fidaxomicin, and several probiotic therapies intended to restore her gut flora. Friends and family poured in support, sharing articles and success stories. One story in particular lit a spark of hope in Anna: a patient who had beaten recurrent *C. diff* with something called a fecal transplant. The idea made her cringe at first—taking stool from a healthy donor and transferring it into the sick patient's colon to reintroduce good bacteria. It sounded like science fiction (or maybe just gross), but the results were astounding. Studies and doctors reported cure rates around 80% to 90% with fecal microbiota transplants (FMT) for patients with multiple *C. diff* recurrences.

In contrast, simply pounding the bacteria with more antibiotics often failed once an infection kept coming back. The healthy microbes from a donor could do what drugs could not: rebuild the gut's natural defense system to crowd out *C. diff* for good.

After her second episode, Anna decided she was willing to try anything. With her physician's referral, she met with a specialist who performed fecal transplants. They walked her through the process—sourcing screened donor stool from a stool bank, and delivering it via a colonoscopy. In early spring, Anna underwent the procedure. It was quick and painless, far easier than all the IVs and hospital stays she'd endured. In the weeks that followed, she noticed a remarkable improvement. Her bowel habits returned to normal completely. The fatigue lifted, and a healthy glow returned to her cheeks. For the first time in months, she felt whole. "FMT may sound weird and gross, but it was the best decision I ever made," she told a friend later, laughing with genuine joy.

Anna was finally free from the *C. diff* cycle. She emerged not only healthier, but wiser, with a new found appreciation for the delicate balance of the human body.

The experience left her passionate about educating others. She shared her story at her community center's health fair, describing how something as simple as a pill for strep throat led to a battle with a dangerous superbug. People listened with rapt attention and horror. Many had never heard of *C. diff*. Anna emphasized that while antibiotics are precious tools, they must be used with care. Every prescription is a double-edged sword—it can cure, but it can also cut the beneficial bacteria that keep us safe. By the end of her talk, a number of folks vowed to think twice and ask their doctors questions like, "Is this antibiotic really necessary?" the next time they had a sniffle or sore throat.

Ms. Jay and Anna Carter's harrowing experiences are far from isolated anecdotes; they are snapshots of a much larger epidemic unfolding in hospitals and homes worldwide. *Clostridioides difficile* infection, once considered a rare complication, has become disturbingly common. In the United States alone, this bacterium causes approximately 500,000 infections every year, and around 30,000 people die as a direct result.

To put it plainly, *C. diff* is one of the deadliest health-care-related infections doctors face today. It preys on the vulnerable moments when our bodies are trying to heal and often strikes in the aftermath of antibiotic use. The two stories in this chapter highlight different faces of the problem: one an older patient in a hospital, and the other a young mother in the community. Together, they illustrate a sobering truth: Antibiotic overuse and misuse are fueling a crisis that spares no one.

How exactly does a drug meant to help us end up causing such harm? The answer lies in the complex ecosystem of the human gut microbiome. Our intestines are home to trillions of bacteria, many of them beneficial. They act as gatekeepers, crowding out invaders and even producing substances that keep the gut lining healthy. When we take antibiotics, especially broad-spectrum ones, we essentially napalm the battlefield—the medication wipes out a wide swath of bacteria, both bad and good. In the aftermath, hardy foes like *C. diff* can survive the onslaught (partly because *C. diff* produces tough spores) and find little competition left. They set up camp in the gut, multiply rapidly, and release toxins that attack the intestinal wall. The result is pseudomembranous colitis, an inflammation of the colon that causes severe diarrhea, abdominal pain, and fever. In extreme cases, the colon can become dangerously enlarged (toxic megacolon) or even perforate, leading to life-threatening complications.

Under a microscope, *C. diff* bacteria look like innocent purple rods with lazy, spaghetti-like tails, but there is nothing innocent about what they do. These germs are uniquely equipped to thrive in the post-antibiotic chaos.

They are resistant to many drugs, and their spores can live on surfaces for months, waiting for a chance to infect a new host.

Once established in a person's gut, *C. diff* is notoriously hard to fully eliminate. The stories of Ms. Jay and Anna showed how recurrences happen all too frequently. In fact, studies show that as many as 35% of patients experience a recurrence after their first *C. diff* infection is treated. And among those who get a second episode, up to 60% may have yet another episode afterward.

This creates a vicious cycle: Each recurrence often means another round of antibiotics (like vancomycin or fidaxomicin) to treat it, which in turn can delay the recovery of healthy gut bacteria and leave the door open for *C. diff* to strike again.

It's a dreadful loop of "cure, recurrence, repeat" that patients and doctors know all too well. The human cost of this infection goes beyond the physical symptoms. Patients endure isolation (since C. diff is contagious, they often will be quarantined in hospitals), embarrassment, and anxiety. It can take a profound psychological toll. Imagine being afraid to eat because you're not sure if it will send you running to the bathroom, or fearing the medicine you need because it might trigger yet another episode. Some survivors, especially after extended battles, develop post-traumatic stress from the experience of severe illness and hospitalization. Others live with long-term consequences, such as irritable bowel syndrome or dietary intolerance, even after the infection is gone. Families are affected too; normal life pauses as loved ones become caregivers, donning gloves and masks, and household routines turn into infection-control drills. The ripple effects of one C. diff case can spread through a whole family and community.

Why has *C. diff* become so prevalent? A major factor is antibiotic overuse in hospitals, clinics, and even on the farm. We now know that a significant fraction of antibiotic prescriptions are unnecessary. The Centers for Disease Control and Prevention (CDC) has found that in hospital settings 30% to 50% of antibiotics prescribed are inappropriate: given for too long, for the wrong condition, or when they aren't needed at all. In outpatient clinics, doctors sometimes prescribe antibiotics for viral illnesses (like the common cold or flu) that antibiotics can't even cure, just to be "safe" or because patients expect a prescription. This well-intentioned misuse does more harm than good.

As one CDC public announcement bluntly stated, treating a viral infection with antibiotics not only won't help; it can make those drugs less effective when you truly need them and raise the risk of *C. diff* infection in the meantime.

C. diff has thrived in this environment of frequent antibiotic exposure. It has also evolved and adapted, with certain strains becoming more virulent (causing more severe illness) and resistant to medications. Around the early 2000s, a hyper-virulent strain emerged that led to outbreaks with higher death rates. Meanwhile, the bacteria's spores lurk in healthcare facilities; if cleaning practices slip or hand hygiene is lacking, *C. diff* finds its next victim. The result of these factors is a pathogen that the CDC has labeled an urgent public health threat, one of the top five most dangerous microbes we face today in the era of antibiotic resistance.

When the Last Patient's Antibiotics Become Your Problem

On a hazy Wednesday in Los Angeles, Maya could see the Hollywood Hills through the hospital window, pale as chalk in the late afternoon. Her new room felt safe. Fresh sheets. Polished rails. That faint citrus-clean smell you notice on every ward from Santa Monica to Pasadena. She was twenty, a college swimmer who spent dawns slicing laps in a campus pool, and Sundays at church playing the piano. She was finally being admitted for the diarrhea that had ambushed her after practice a week earlier. At first, she blamed the bad takeout fried rice she ate with her relay team. No one else got sick. She was the only one sprinting to the bathroom every hour, cramping and weak.

At urgent care, she was dehydrated, a bag of IV fluid made her feel briefly human, and then everything slid again. She was desperate and sent a text to her prayer partners, asking them to pray for her. Stool tests told the real story: *C. difficile.* She started oral vancomycin, and the tide slowly turned. Two weeks later, she was back on her feet and ready to go home.

There was one part that made no sense to her. She had not taken antibiotics in years. No recent dental work, no over-the-counter medications, and no prescriptions. Her only brush with a hospital had been ten days before the diarrhea started, an overnight stay for rhabdomyolysis (muscle breakdown) after a brutal dryland workout in the valley heat. A few bags of fluid fixed her kidneys, and she was discharged the next morning. No antibiotics. No obvious risk. Her doctors were glad she was better, but they could not explain why this had happened.

What Maya could not see in that spotless room was the fingerprint of the patient who had slept there before her. *C. difficile* spreads by spores that cling to surfaces and survive ordinary cleaning. When someone receives antibiotics, their protective gut bacteria are knocked down, *C. diff* finds space to bloom, and trillions of hardy spores ride out into the world on hands, rails, call buttons, floors, and bedside tables. The room can look perfect and still carry a shadow.

A large study asked a simple unsettling question: Does it matter what happened to the person who used your hospital bed before you? It turned out the answer was YES!

Researchers looked at patients admitted to hospital rooms and compared two groups:

- People whose prior bed occupant had received antibiotics
- People whose prior bed occupant had not received antibiotics

The patients themselves were otherwise similar in age, health, and underlying conditions. Even after adjusting for all of that, the people who followed someone who had been on antibiotics were about 40% more likely to develop *C. diff* infection.

To make that more concrete: Over the first fourteen days in the hospital, about four out of every thousand patients in "clean ancestry" beds (no antibiotics in the prior occupant) got *C. diff*. That number jumped to about seven out of every thousand when the previous occupant had been given antibiotics. The only thing that changed was what happened to a stranger days earlier in the same room.

That extra risk showed up even in patients who never swallowed a single dose of antibiotics themselves. The room's history becomes part of their story.

This "room effect" has been confirmed in other studies as well. In one analysis, patients admitted to rooms where a previous occupant had *C. diff* had higher chances of getting

C. diff themselves. The odds increased by about 27% if they entered that room within ninety days, and by roughly 40% if the exposure was within a year. Another study used real-time location tracking and found that simply lying in a contaminated bed was associated with about a 50% higher odds of hospital-onset *C. diff.*

Think of a busy medical floor: Doors open and close. Teams round. Housekeeping works hard, yet cannot eliminate every spore as antibiotics reshape the ward's invisible biology. In that sense, antibiotics behave a bit like secondhand smoke. Your personal risk is shaped not only by what you are given, but by how much antibiotic "smoke" is in the air around you, on the bed rails and bathroom tiles you share with strangers.

When Maya's medical team traced the details, they learned that the last patient in her bed had received a long course of IV antibiotics for a heart infection. It was nobody's fault in the simple sense.

That person needed treatment. The room was cleaned. The staff followed the rules. Yet biology kept its own score. Spores outlasted the mop, and a swimmer from the South Bay carried the bill.

This is why stewardship is not a lecture about saying no. It is a practical way to make rooms safer for the next patient who rolls into bed N314 at dusk. The fewer and narrower the antibiotics we use, the lower the background pressure of *C. diff* on a unit. The more often we reach for soap, water, and sporicidal wipes, the less likely it is that a clean bed will hide *C. diff* spores. These choices are quiet and cumulative. They protect the one patient in front of us and the unseen patient who follows.

Maya healed. The vancomycin and prayers worked. She walked out into a Westside evening that smelled faintly of jasmine and car exhaust. She was grateful. Weeks later, she eased back into the pool, counting strokes and breathing every third, unhurried for once.

She now knows that hospitals keep two kinds of histories. The one written in charts. And the one written on surfaces by the antibiotics we use. Both can shape a life.

Fighting back with hope

Yet amid the urgency of this crisis, there is also hope and progress. The medical community is fighting back on multiple fronts to ensure stories like those of Ms. Jay and Anna become rarer. Prevention is front and center. Since most C. diff infections are triggered by antibiotics or occur in healthcare settings, targeted efforts can make a big difference. Here are some key strategies being employed:

- Improving antibiotic stewardship: Hospitals and clinics are implementing programs to ensure antibiotics are used only when necessary and correctly. This means doctors are being more cautious about prescribing broad-spectrum drugs, opting for targeted therapies or alternative treatments when possible. Patients are also being educated to understand that antibiotics aren't a cure-all—for example, a viral sore throat won't benefit from them. Studies suggest that cutting unnecessary antibiotic use by even a modest amount might significantly reduce C. diff infection rates. Every antibiotic prescription that is avoided when it isn't absolutely needed is one less opportunity for C. diff to take hold.

- Stringent infection control: Healthcare facilities have stepped up protocols to halt the spread of C. diff spores. This includes rigorous cleaning of rooms with sporicidal disinfectants (bleach-based cleaners that can kill *C. diff* spores), ultraviolet-C light disinfection, isolating infected patients, and using protective gowns and gloves for anyone entering their room. Proper hand-washing (with soap and water, since alcohol sanitizers don't kill *C. diff* spores) is non-negotiable for staff, patients, and visitors alike. These measures help break the chain of transmission, so one patient's illness doesn't become an outbreak.

- Protecting vulnerable patients: Extra care is given to those at high risk, such as older adults or people with serious illnesses who are on antibiotics. Doctors may choose shorter antibiotic courses or add probiotics (beneficial bacteria) in some cases to help maintain gut flora (though probiotics are not a guaranteed shield; some evidence suggests they might lower the risk of *C. diff* in certain scenarios). Hospitals are also flagging patients with a history of *C. diff* so that if they are admitted, precautions can start immediately.

These are not entirely new strategies; they have been tested and proven and demand our consistent use. In the early 2000s, when the hyper-virulent *C. diff* strain NAP1/027 was ravaging hospitals and killing patients, England took a bold step. They didn't treat *C. diff* as a routine hospital nuisance. They treated it like a ward fire that kept reigniting, and responded with a national, all-hands playbook. Starting in April 2007, National Health Service (NHS) acute trusts had to report *C. diff* cases every month, so the problem couldn't be hidden in local spreadsheets or explained away as "just bad luck." Around the same time, they built the *Clostridioides difficile* Ribotyping Network (the CDRN) to spot and track the more virulent strains, including the epidemic ribotype 027, so outbreaks could be recognized early and addressed with real precision.

Then came accountability with teeth. England set a national reduction target (often cited as a 30% cut over three years) and tied it to performance management and financial penalties for missing the mark. But the move that helped change the biology of the battlefield was stewardship: Hospitals deliberately pulled back on the antibiotics most likely to fuel *C. diff*, especially fluoroquinolones (and also cephalosporins), lowering the "selective pressure" that had given 027 an edge.

Large analyses of the decline in England found that fluoroquinolone restriction best explained the sharp drop.

At the bedside, the guidance was equally blunt and practical: isolate quickly, use gloves and aprons, prioritize soap-and-water handwashing because alcohol gel doesn't kill spores well, and perform daily and terminal cleaning with effective decontamination. England even launched a government-funded NHS "Deep Clean" drive to restore ward cleanliness during the peak period. The payoff was dramatic: After the mid-2000s peak, England's *C. diff* incidence fell by roughly 80% after 2006, and the data point again and again to stewardship, especially fluoroquinolone restriction, as the key lever that helped the epidemic strain lose its advantage.

At the same time, research and innovation are providing new tools to treat *C. diff* and prevent its return. We saw how fecal microbiota transplantation offered a dramatic cure for Anna when antibiotics alone failed. For years, FMT was considered an experimental, last-resort therapy—and it was literally done by transferring donor stool in blended solutions. But now, science has taken that concept and refined it. In a groundbreaking move, the FDA approved two therapeutics (in late 2022 and early 2023) designed to prevent *C. diff* from recurring by restoring healthy gut bacteria. These are essentially standardized, purified forms of fecal transplant in a more palatable package (one is given as an enema, another as oral capsules). This development is a game-changer: It takes the success of an old "folk" remedy and transforms it into an officially sanctioned medication. As one infectious disease expert said, "The future is here." After years of racing to find better solutions, we finally have approved therapies that break the cycle of recurrence by healing the microbiome instead of hammering it with more antibiotics. These treatments are becoming more widely available, bringing new hope to patients who have suffered multiple *C. diff* bouts

Researchers are also working on other fronts, including vaccines to prevent *C. diff* infection (several are in trials) and novel non-antibiotic drugs that neutralize the *C. diff* toxins. The battle against *C. diff* is becoming smarter and more empathetic, focusing not just on killing a bacterium, but on caring for the whole patient, gut flora and all.

Perhaps one of the most hopeful signs is the change in mindset happening among healthcare professionals and patients alike. The stories of Ms. Jay and Anna Carter underscore a crucial lesson: We cannot take antibiotics for granted. The medical community is increasingly treating antibiotics as a precious resource—one to be preserved and respected. Public awareness campaigns urge people to "Get Smart About Antibiotics," emphasizing that these drugs are not needed for every sniffle, and improper use can have grave consequences. Patients are learning to ask questions, and doctors are thinking twice. This culture shift, though gradual, will be key to turning the tide. After all, *C. diff* is essentially a preventable infection. If we prevent the reckless overuse of antibiotics and uphold rigorous hygiene, we can stop many cases before they ever begin. Each prevention is a victory; a life not disrupted, a story like Ms. Jay's not repeated.

As we close this chapter on *C. diff*, it's clear that our relationship with antibiotics is complicated. These drugs have saved countless lives, including likely Ms. Jay's and Anna's at different points, yet they nearly took those same lives in a roundabout way. It's a reminder that in medicine, every action has consequences, sometimes far beyond our foresight. The gut feeling we all must develop is one of cautious optimism. We should appreciate antibiotics, but also respect their power and use them wisely. By doing so, we honor the hard lessons learned through stories like these and move toward a future where healing does not come at such a high cost.

Same Medicine, Different Salt

Not every gut problem is a microbiome problem. Sometimes the trouble starts higher up, in the narrow corridor of the esophagus, where the way a pill dissolves can make all the difference. On a crisp October afternoon in the Berkshires, the maples along Route 7 were showing off. A twenty-four-year-old named Rowan Hale and a few friends followed a ridge trail near Mount Greylock, took photos above the Housatonic, and joked about who packed the worst trail mix snack. Somewhere between the overlook and the trailhead, a tick found the back of Rowan's knee. He couldn't tell how long the tick had been there, as this was their third day hiking. He flicked it away, thought nothing of it, and kept moving.

By January, his right knee had ballooned. It felt warm, tight, and stubborn. Rowan tried to push through with ice and an elastic wrap. When climbing the stairs started to feel like lifting a sandbag, he saw his primary care clinician. The story, the exam, and the tests lined up with Lyme arthritis that had smoldered since that fall hike.

He left with a prescription for doxycycline hyclate. It is the version most pharmacies carry, easy to find, and usually a little cheaper, so it tends to be the default for short courses in this part of Massachusetts. Rowan also has a history of reflux disease, which he has battled with over-the-counter antacids. He took his first dose late at night with a quick sip of water and went to sleep. By morning, he was nauseated. Day two brought vomiting and a raw, burning stripe behind his breastbone. He tried crackers and ginger tea. He tried powering through. Within a week, he had lost weight and looked like someone who was sick of being sick.

At a local hospital clinic, an infectious diseases specialist listened to the whole timeline and nodded. "Same antibiotic, two common salts," she said. "Hyclate is the one you were given. It can dissolve in a way that's rough on the esophagus, especially if you already have reflux or take it right before bed. There is another salt called monohydrate that many people find gentler on the stomach. They both fight Lyme well if you can keep them down. "

They switched him to doxycycline monohydrate and changed the routine: *Take every pill with a full glass of water. Take it during the day, not at bedtime. Stay upright for at least thirty minutes after each dose. A small snack is fine if it helps your stomach. Take antacids, calcium, magnesium, iron, and multivitamins at least a couple of hours before or after the pill, since those minerals can bind to the medicine and blunt its effect.*

Rowan felt wary. "Why don't we start with the gentler one if it exists? "

"Because hyclate is everywhere," the specialist said. "Most people tolerate it; it comes in more strengths and forms, and it usually costs a bit less out of pocket. For someone without reflux or a history of pill irritation, it is a practical first choice. When nausea or heartburn gets in the way, we adjust. In longer treatments, like for acne or rosacea, we often begin with monohydrate for comfort over the long haul. "

Within forty-eight hours of the switch, the nausea eased. By the end of the week, his appetite had returned. The knee stopped feeling like a hot drum and started acting like a joint again. He finished the course, kept his follow-up, and went back to short hikes with permethrin-treated socks and careful tick checks.

On his last clinic visit, the specialist summarized what had happened, not as a lecture but as a recipe Rowan could remember. "The drug did not change, only the salt and the way you take it. Hyclate is the common, convenient option and works well for most.

Monohydrate can be kinder to the upper GI tract because it is less acidic when it dissolves, which matters when reflux is part of your story or when treatment will last. Either one needs space from minerals, an upright body, and enough water to keep the pill moving. "

Rowan laughed about the worst trail mix again, this time with a lighter step. The knee was quiet, the weight was back, and the lesson felt simple and practical. The right medicine is sometimes the same medicine, taken in a way your body can live with.

As the next chapter will explore, the burden of antibiotic-related problems doesn't stop at gut-wrenching infections.

In fact, another equally alarming issue is growing: allergic reactions to antibiotics. From mild skin rashes that itch and annoy, to sudden bouts of swelling and difficulty breathing, and even to the terrifying collapse of anaphylactic shock, patients are experiencing allergies to the very drugs meant to cure them. These allergic reactions are increasing and pose their own puzzles and perils. How can a "miracle drug" turn into a lethal threat inside someone's body? What do we do when the cure itself makes us sick? In Chapter 3: "Allergic to the Cure," we will uncover why more people are becoming allergic to antibiotics, how this trend further complicates the healing process, and what can be done to protect patients from reactions ranging from inconvenient to life-threatening. The tale of antibiotics is far from over, and with each chapter, we get closer to understanding how to truly go *beyond the cure.*

Key ideas
- Antibiotics disrupt the microbiome, triggering C. difficile.
- Narrow-spectrum and shorter courses disturb less.
- Food, fiber, and time help recovery.
- If you develop new watery diarrhea (especially with fever or blood), call! Or go to the emergency room! Don't self-treat.

Do this — Readers
- Take antibiotics only when there is a clear bacterial need; finish the agreed course.
- Ask if a narrower option or shorter duration is appropriate.

- Ask about how to take the pills, with or without food, and what to avoid.

Do this — Clinicians
- Default to the narrowest effective agent and the shortest evidence-based duration.
- Flag C. diff risk (age, prior antibiotic use, prior C. diff episodes, proton-pump inhibitor use); provide return precautions.
- Document indication, duration, and reassess at forty-eight to seventy-two hours.

Conversation starters
- "Is there a narrower antibiotic or a shorter course that would work for me?"
- "What should I watch for that could mean C. diff?"

For the everyday side effects that push people to quit early or self-treat, see the Bonus Chapter: "Small Harms, Big Consequences." You can also visit the book website at *Beyondthecurebook.com*

<h1 style="text-align:center">Chapter 3</h1>

Allergic to the Cure

Writing about allergic reactions has always felt personal. Before my close friend's son, Kofi Asante, was born, I didn't fully grasp the complex web of emotional, social, and medical challenges that allergies weave into daily life. Kofi's story, shared with his parents' permission, changed that. It made me see allergies not as inconveniences, but as life-altering conditions that demand constant vigilance.

From his earliest days, Kofi seemed to be at odds with food. As a newborn, he battled stubborn rashes, colic, and discomfort whenever his parents tried to supplement breastfeeding with formula or other types of milk. Every new attempt ended in the same way: tears, irritated skin, restless nights. His parents, both physicians, approached the problem with the determination they brought to their medical work, but nothing seemed to bring relief.

By the time he turned three, Kofi had developed a careful, almost wary relationship with food. His older brother ate freely, enjoying everything from fruit to pasta, but Kofi's approach was cautious. Meals were less about enjoyment and more about survival, shaped by painful past experiences. His restricted diet worried his parents, who knew he wasn't getting the variety he needed.

One morning, hoping to expand his nutrition, Kofi's father offered him a small bite of cooked egg white, rich in protein and nutrients. Within minutes, the calm morning turned into chaos. Kofi began vomiting violently, coughing, and growing frighteningly limp.

In that moment, his medically trained parents weren't doctors; they were terrified parents watching their child's body rebel.

Thankfully, he stabilized by the next day. The message was clear: Eggs weren't just unwelcome; they were dangerous.

A year later, it happened again. It was a sunny Sunday, and Kofi's mother had made peanut soup, a beloved Ghanaian dish. This version used peanut butter paste, a substitute for the fresh groundnuts used back home. Everyone was enjoying the meal, but Kofi hesitated. His father encouraged him to try a small spoonful. Kofi shook his head and pulled away, but a drop of soup brushed his lip and arm. Within minutes, his lip swelled, and hives erupted where the soup had touched his skin. His parents' minds raced with the frightening thought of what could have happened if he had swallowed more.

Formal allergy testing confirmed their fears: Kofi was severely allergic to egg whites, peanuts, and seafood. From then on, an epinephrine auto-injector was never out of reach. It became a quiet but constant presence, a lifeline, and a reminder of how thin the line is between safety and crisis.

Kofi's allergies reshaped every corner of his family's life. They learned that allergies aren't small inconveniences; they're life-defining. They turn simple meals and common medications into potential threats. And while food allergies might seem far removed from medication allergies, the underlying cause is often the same: an immune system that mistakes the harmless for the dangerous.

When most people think of allergies, they picture spring pollen, shellfish, or peanut allergies. But antibiotics? These medical miracles, hailed as lifesaving achievements, can also carry hidden hazards. Each year, more than 1.3 million people in the United States end up in emergency rooms because of medication-related allergic reactions, and antibiotics lead the list. In children, they account for up to half of all medication-induced allergic visits to pediatric ERs. Behind every number is a family suddenly thrown into panic, watching hives spread across a child's skin, or hearing the desperate sound of someone struggling to breathe.

These reactions range from mild rashes to rare but severe crises. A small number of people develop severe cutaneous adverse reactions (or SCARs). These are uncommon, but they're emergencies because they can worsen quickly. Two examples should be known by name: SJS/TEN (Stevens-Johnson syndrome/toxic epidermal necrolysis) and DRESS.

SJS/TEN often starts with fever, sore throat, and a rapidly spreading rash that may become painful or involve the mouth, eyes, or genitals.

DRESS (drug reaction with eosinophilia and systemic symptoms) can show up later, often two to eight weeks after starting a drug, with rash plus fever, sometimes facial swelling, swollen glands, and signs that internal organs (especially liver or kidneys) are being affected.

If you develop a new widespread rash with fever, skin pain, or mouth or eye involvement while taking an antibiotic, stop the medication and seek urgent medical care the same day. Do not "push through." Do not restart the drug unless a clinician explicitly tells you it's safe.

Anaphylaxis can close off the airway in minutes. And even when patients survive, the scars—physical and emotional—can be permanent. For doctors, these cases create lasting challenges, too. A single "allergic" label can limit treatment options for years, forcing the use of less effective or more toxic drugs at a time when antibiotic resistance is already a growing global threat.

The challenge is that many people labeled as allergic, especially to penicillin, aren't truly allergic at all. Studies show that more than 90% of those with a penicillin allergy label can tolerate the drug after testing. Sometimes the original reaction was a mild rash unrelated to the drug, or a childhood event that no longer poses a risk. Yet the label persists, influencing treatment choices decades later. And an allergy to one antibiotic does not automatically mean you're allergic to all related antibiotics—what matters is the specific drug and the type of reaction.

These incorrect labels have a ripple effect. They push doctors toward broad-spectrum antibiotics, powerful but less precise weapons that fuel resistance. That's why hospitals and clinics are working to confirm or remove false allergy labels. Careful history-taking, allergy testing, and updated records don't just improve individual care; they also help preserve antibiotics for the future.

Kofi's story shows us how real allergies alter lives, and how easily false ones can complicate care. Whether it's a peanut hidden in a favorite family recipe or penicillin prescribed for an infection, allergies reveal the delicate nature of our immune system. And they remind us that every label, every prescription, and every dose carries weight.

When Harold's body turned against him

Harold Blackstone was sixty-seven, a retired school principal with a sharp mind and a fiercely independent spirit. A recent hip fracture had forced him into a rehabilitation center, a change he found difficult but necessary if he wanted to walk without pain again.

For a while, his recovery seemed steady, until one afternoon when everything shifted. Harold became confused, unable to follow conversations. His temperature climbed. Concerned staff called 9-1-1, and by the time the ambulance arrived, his disorientation had deepened. He could no longer give his own medical history.

In the emergency department, the physician took in the facts: fever, confusion, and a positive urinalysis suggesting a urinary tract infection. It was a common pattern in elderly patients, especially those coming from nursing homes or rehab facilities. The logical next step seemed clear. Ceftriaxone, a broad-spectrum antibiotic frequently used for UTIs, was ordered and started through an IV.

But almost immediately, Harold's body turned against him. His heart began to race. His blood pressure dropped. His throat tightened until he could barely draw a breath. Alarms sounded as the medical team rushed to his side. Epinephrine was pushed in an effort to halt the severe allergic reaction. His pulse faded, and for a few terrifying moments, his heart stopped. Chest compressions began. Oxygen flowed. More medications were given. Slowly, a faint pulse returned.

Harold was moved to the ICU, where he spent several days under close watch. As his condition stabilized, the truth came into focus. The rehab center had documented a severe allergy to ceftriaxone in his chart, but that detail had never been included in the paperwork sent with him. One missing line had nearly cost him his life.

And there was more. The initial diagnosis that had set this chain of events in motion—the presumed urinary tract infection—was wrong. Further imaging and cultures revealed something far more dangerous: MRSA discitis and osteomyelitis, a resistant strain of Staphylococcus aureus infecting the discs and bones in his spine. The urinalysis findings that had seemed convincing were incidental, a red herring that often misleads in elderly patients.

Once the correct diagnosis was made, ceftriaxone was stopped, and Harold was started on vancomycin, the right antibiotic for MRSA. Over the next five weeks, he endured a long course of treatment and physical therapy before finally returning home.

But recovery brought more than physical healing. Harold and his family were left with the sobering realization that he had almost died, not from his actual illness, but from a preventable mistake. A simple phone call to the rehab facility could have revealed his allergy before the first dose was given. A more cautious approach to diagnosis could have avoided treating the wrong infection entirely.

Harold's case is a reminder of two critical truths in medicine: Allergies must be verified, and assumptions can kill. While urinary tract infections are common in older adults, they are not the cause of every fever or episode of confusion. Careful history-taking and confirmation of the facts are not luxuries. They are the very foundation of safe care.

A devastating outcome

Amanda Reed was twenty-six, a graduate student who seemed to carry sunlight with her wherever she went. She thrived in her environmental science program, as comfortable hiking a rugged trail as she was buried in research data. Friends admired her energy and curiosity, qualities that made her feel unstoppable.

That summer, in the second year of her program, a simple urinary tract infection set her on a path she could never have imagined. It began with the usual discomfort: urgency, burning, a fever that wouldn't break. At the urgent care clinic, the doctor prescribed trimethoprim-sulfamethoxazole, better known as Bactrim. It was a routine choice, one she had taken in the past without trouble. Amanda filled the prescription without hesitation, expecting little more than some mild stomach upset.

By the third day, something felt off. She was exhausted in a way that seemed deeper than the infection. Her skin itched. A faint rash appeared on her arms. She brushed it off as heat rash or a reaction to laundry detergent, but by evening, the rash had spread across her chest and back. Her lips cracked and bled. Her eyes grew red and swollen. Blisters began forming on her hands, and the pain became unbearable.

Her roommate drove her to the emergency room. The doctors took one look and knew she was in danger. Amanda was diagnosed with Stevens–Johnson syndrome, a rare but devastating reaction to certain medications, including antibiotics like Bactrim. In SJS, the immune system turns against the body, attacking skin and mucous membranes. What begins as a rash can escalate into layers of skin blistering and peeling away, leaving raw tissue exposed and vulnerable to infection.

She was transferred to the burn unit for intensive care. Treating SJS is as demanding as treating severe burns. Her skin had to be cleaned and dressed daily to prevent infection. Pain was constant. Her care team worked to stabilize her, but the open wounds became infected. The inflammation overwhelmed her organs.

Her parents stayed at her bedside, watching the vibrant daughter they knew fade into a fragile figure wrapped in dressings. Five days after her admission, Amanda's heart stopped. The doctors tried to revive her, but the infection had spread too far. She was gone, her future erased by a reaction so rare and cruel it left everyone reeling.

Her death left behind difficult questions. Had Bactrim been the best choice for her UTI? Could a different antibiotic, or even delayed treatment, have changed the outcome? While antibiotics like Bactrim are highly effective, they are not without risk, especially for non-life-threatening infections.

The link between antibiotics and severe reactions like SJS underscores a delicate balance. These drugs are among the greatest medical achievements in history, but their misuse and overuse increase the chances of rare yet catastrophic outcomes. Amanda had no reason to suspect that a medication she had tolerated before could suddenly turn deadly.

Antibiotic overuse doesn't just breed resistant bacteria. It can prime the immune system to overreact, doubling the risk of developing an allergy with each unnecessary course. In children, early antibiotic use can alter immune development, raising the risk not only of antibiotic allergies but also of food and environmental allergies later in life.

Their immune systems can become hypersensitive, like a smoke alarm that triggers at the faintest trace of smoke or even without smoke at all.

Why do these allergic reactions occur at all? The immune system is usually skilled at distinguishing harmful invaders from harmless substances. But sometimes it misfires, mistaking a medication for a threat. This sets off a cascade of immune chemicals—histamines and others—that can cause anything from mild rashes to life-threatening anaphylaxis. Reactions can be immediate or delayed, appearing days or even weeks later, as in Stevens–Johnson syndrome.

Genetics can make some people more susceptible. Prior exposure to a drug can "prime" the immune system for a stronger response on subsequent encounters.

Viral infections, prolonged use, and even the way a medication is given can increase the risk.

The most troubling part is how unpredictable these reactions are. A drug that was tolerated before can suddenly trigger an allergy. And once that label is applied, it can shape a patient's medical future in ways that are hard to undo.

Amanda's story is a reminder of the balance medicine must strike: Antibiotics save lives, but they also carry real risks. It is a call for thoughtful prescribing, careful monitoring, and the understanding that no medication is without potential harm.

The impact of antibiotics does not stop with the immune system. Just as they can provoke deadly allergic reactions, they can also damage other vital organs. In the next chapter, War on the Kidneys, we will see how the very drugs designed to heal can silently injure the body's filtration system, and the human cost of that hidden battle.

Key ideas

- Many "penicillin allergies" aren't true allergies and limit good options.
- True immediate allergies can be life-threatening; know the signs.
- Delabeling improves care.

Do this — Readers

- Write down what happened, how soon, and how it was treated.
- If your "allergy" was a remote rash or upset stomach, ask about testing or delabeling.
- Know emergency signs—hives, swelling, breathing trouble—and seek urgent care.

Do this — Clinicians

- Take a structured allergy history; consider test dosing or referral.
- Use cross-reactivity evidence to expand options safely.
- Update the chart after delabeling.

Conversation starters

- "Can we review whether my penicillin 'allergy' is real?"
- "Is delabeling safe for me?"

Chapter 4
War on the Kidneys

lex Carter could still smell the tang of disinfectant. It lingered in the back of his throat as he lay under the harsh hospital lights. A week ago, he had been unstoppable. Twenty-eight years old. A weightlifter who could hoist twice his body weight. The kind of man who thought discipline could outmatch anything.

Now his body felt foreign. His legs were swollen. His skin was dry. His mouth was painfully parched. Tubes snaked from his arms into beeping machines. The numbers on the screen told the truth faster than words. His kidneys were in trouble.

Blood tests confirmed what the monitor hinted at: The organs that had quietly filtered his blood every second of his life were faltering. It didn't make sense. He hadn't been sick in years. The only problem, as far as he knew, was a small cut on his shin from a dropped weight plate. He had brushed it off. But the scrape grew hot and angry. By the time he limped into urgent care, the bacteria had the upper hand.

The antibiotic felt like salvation. "Vancomycin," the nurse said with quiet confidence. And it was a hero. The kind summoned when all others failed. The weapon of choice against MRSA, a bacterium notorious for resisting weaker drugs. Within days, his fever broke. The pain in his leg faded. Alex thought the worst was over.

But vancomycin carries a shadow. It is both a lifesaver and a saboteur. It can win the battle while quietly waging a second war against the body. Its origin story reads like a page from a medical adventure novel: In 1952, a missionary in the jungles of Borneo sent a scoop of soil to a scientist friend at Eli Lilly.

That soil contained a microorganism that produced a compound capable of "vanquishing" stubborn infections that penicillin couldn't touch.

The new drug was named vancomycin (think "vanquish"), and by 1958, it was approved for use. Early batches of vancomycin were notoriously impure, a brownish cocktail nicknamed "Mississippi mud," and patients who received those doses sometimes suffered alarming side effects, including kidney damage and hearing loss. Because of those toxic effects, for decades vancomycin was held back as a last-resort antibiotic, something to be used only when absolutely necessary.

Over the years, pharmaceutical advances have purified vancomycin (today's vials are over 90% pure active ingredient), drastically reducing the early-day impurities. The drug earned a safer reputation and became a staple in hospitals, especially as MRSA and other resistant bacteria spread worldwide. In fact, the rise of antibiotic-resistant infections like MRSA has increased global reliance on vancomycin. The World Health Organization notes that as MRSA became common in hospitals around the world, doctors turned more and more to "last resort" drugs like vancomycin to treat these infections. Vancomycin use is now widespread; it's among the most commonly prescribed hospital antibiotics for serious infections. In Alex's case, vancomycin was the apparent choice to battle the aggressive MRSA in his leg.

Alex didn't know that in the tiny corridors of his kidneys, the drug was causing damage. His urine slowed to a trickle. The scale showed sudden weight gain, not from muscle but from trapped fluid. His muscles felt heavy. Blood work confirmed the worst. His creatinine, a waste product that healthy kidneys clear without effort, had more than doubled. In the fight to save his leg, something else was being lost.

To understand why, you have to know the quiet brilliance of the kidneys. Two fist-size, bean-shaped organs. Resting under the ribs, working without pause. Every drop of blood you own passes through them dozens of times a day. Inside each kidney are nearly a million filtration units called nephrons. They strain, sift, and fine-tune, deciding in moments what to keep and what to discard. They balance electrolytes. They regulate blood pressure. They keep you alive without asking for recognition, until they can't.

The tragedy is that the very drugs meant to save life can sometimes harm these guardians. Vancomycin's kidney toxicity is well known. Depending on dose, duration, and the patient, anywhere from 5% to 43% of those treated develop kidney injury. Most recover. Some are left with lasting scars. For a few, like Alex, the damage announces itself suddenly, pulling them into a different fight altogether.

Why does vancomycin hurt the kidneys?

Scientists think it targets the proximal tubule cells. These are the hardest-working cells in the nephron. They pull nutrients back into the blood and concentrate the urine. Under the microscope, vancomycin damage often resembles acute tubular necrosis, or ATN. That means some of those cells get injured and die.

Sometimes the drug triggers a different attack, an allergic-type inflammation called acute interstitial nephritis, or AIN. In both cases, the result is the same. The kidneys' filtering slows. Toxins build up. It's a bitter twist: The medicine meant to cure you starts poisoning the very filters designed to clear poisons from your blood.

Most patients never feel it happening. The kidneys are silent fighters. They can take hits for days before showing signs of trouble. Often, the first clue is a blood test that comes back with bad news. Some things make this "friendly fire" more likely.

High doses or long courses. The more vancomycin you get, the greater the risk. At daily doses above four grams, studies have seen kidney injury in more than a third of patients.

Other kidney-harming drugs. Pairing vancomycin with certain antibiotics or other nephrotoxic medicines can be like a one-two punch. Piperacillin-tazobactam, for example, can multiply the risk.

Patient factors. Dehydration, preexisting kidney disease, obesity, and advanced age can all tip the balance. In Alex's case, his muscular build meant his creatinine was already on the high side. His protein-heavy diet and supplement use may have left him borderline dehydrated. That gave vancomycin an easier target.

After a week on the drug, Alex's kidneys gave up. His doctors stopped the vancomycin and switched to a different antibiotic. They pushed fluids. Slowly, his numbers began to improve. Youth and fitness were on his side. Two weeks later, his kidneys were working again. But the episode left a mark. For Alex and his medical team, it was proof of how thin the line can be between saving a life and harming it.

That's why vancomycin dosing is a tightrope. Too little, and the infection wins. Too much, and the kidneys take the blow. For decades, doctors used "trough levels," the lowest drug concentration before the next dose, as their guide. They aimed for fifteen to twenty micrograms per milliliter for serious infections. It seemed safe.

But newer research showed that high troughs can mean unnecessary drug exposure. And with that, higher toxicity.

In 2020, the Infectious Diseases Society of America changed the rules. The new target is no longer just a trough number. It's the AUC—the area under the concentration-time curve.

In plain terms, it measures the drug's total exposure over time. For MRSA, the sweet spot is an AUC of 400 to 600 mg·hr/L: High enough to kill bacteria. Low enough to protect the kidneys. Modern technology makes this possible. Pharmacists now use software to crunch patient-specific data. One approach, Bayesian dosing, blends population models with an individual's drug levels to predict the best dose. With just one vancomycin level from Alex, a program could have adjusted his dosing to hit the target without overshooting. Some hospital systems even flag dangerous drug levels before the damage starts.

Still, the simplest protection is to use vancomycin only when it's truly needed. That's where antibiotic stewardship comes in. Many hospitals now check culture results quickly and switch patients to safer drugs if MRSA isn't confirmed. This avoids unnecessary exposure and unnecessary risk.

Alex was lucky. He walked out of the hospital with both his kidneys and his leg intact. His doctors gave him the same advice they give many patients: stay hydrated and keep an eye on kidney function if you're on strong antibiotics.

He stepped into the sunlight, thinking the fight was over. It wasn't. Another kidney war was raging worldwide. A quieter one. This time, the enemy was crystal.

Stones in the Water: A Growing Epidemic

While Alex was fighting a sudden, drug-induced kidney injury, millions of others are battling a slower enemy. Kidney stones.

They've been with us for millennia. Even Egyptian mummies have them. For decades, stones were mostly an adult problem. Men in their forties or fifties. Often dehydrated. Often living on rich diets.

But that's changing. Stones are showing up in teenagers, even in children. In the United States, rates have jumped by about 70% over the last thirty years. Pediatric urology clinics are calling it an epidemic. Worldwide, the numbers are climbing, too. In 2021, there were more than 100 million new cases. That's up more than a quarter since 2000.

A kidney stone is, at its core, a crystal. It forms when minerals and salts in urine clump together. The most common type is calcium oxalate. Calcium is in our diet. Oxalate is in foods like spinach, nuts, and tea. In the right conditions, they bind, layer by layer, until they become a stone.

Some stones are no bigger than a grain of sand. Others grow to the size of an olive. Small stones may pass unnoticed. Bigger ones can scrape the urinary tract, cause bleeding, and block urine flow. The pain, renal colic, is often described as worse than childbirth.

Why the surge? Doctors point to several culprits.
Dehydration. Many people simply don't drink enough water.
Busy days. Hotter climates. Children on the sports field or in front of screens may ignore thirst until it's too late.
Diet. The "Western diet" is high in salt, animal protein, and sugary drinks. All of these shift urine chemistry toward stone formation. Ironically, too little dietary calcium can also raise the risk.
Obesity. Rising body weight parallels rising stone rates.
Genetics and illness. Family history matters. So do conditions like bowel disease or frequent urinary infections. And then there's a newer suspect. Antibiotics. Especially in childhood.

The Antibiotic–Stone Connection

In 2018, Dr. Gregory Tasian and his team at the Children's Hospital of Philadelphia uncovered a striking link. They reviewed the health records of over 13 million people in the UK. More than 26,000 people had kidney stones.

The question: Had they taken antibiotics beforehand? The answer was yes, and often.

Five classes of antibiotics increased the odds of stones. Sulfa drugs more than doubled the risk. Cephalosporins raised it by nearly 90%. Fluoroquinolones by 67%. Even broad-spectrum penicillins increased the risk by over 20%.

The effect was most substantial in children and teens. Risk peaked in the months after antibiotic use, then slowly declined, but it stayed elevated for years.

Why? The answer may lie in the gut.

Our intestines are home to trillions of bacteria. Some of them, like *Oxalobacter formigenes*, break down oxalate in food. Less oxalate in the gut means less in the urine and fewer stones.

Antibiotics can wipe these helpers out. Especially broad-spectrum ones. The infection is cured. But the gut is left without its oxalate eaters. More oxalate makes it to the kidneys. More crystals form.

A child may take antibiotics for an ear infection at age seven. At seventeen, they could be doubled over in pain from their first kidney stone.

This adds a new dimension to antibiotic stewardship. We already know overuse fuels resistant "superbugs." Now we see it may also fuel an epidemic of stones.

Globally, the same patterns are emerging. Hot climates have long had higher rates of kidney stones caused by dehydration.

But now, as Western diets spread and obesity rises, so do stones. Pediatric cases are appearing in places where they were once unheard of.

Doctors are responding. Hydration campaigns. Diet counseling. Even research into restoring oxalate-eating bacteria to high-risk patients. And always, the reminder: Prescribe antibiotics only when they're truly needed.

The Next Front

Alex's kidneys recovered. He's back in the gym. But he now knows the cost of certain cures.

On the other side of the world, a girl who once suffered kidney stones now drinks extra water and avoids unnecessary antibiotics.

The war on the kidneys can be fought. But it's not the only battlefield.

In the next chapter, "Rhythms of the Heart," we'll leave the kidneys and turn to the heart and ask another unsettling question. Can antibiotics disrupt its rhythm? The answer will take us into stories of sudden arrhythmias and unexpected danger. The war on our organs continues.

Key ideas

- Aminoglycosides, vancomycin, and other drugs can injure the kidneys. The risk rises with dehydration and other nephrotoxins.
- Dosing must match kidney function.

Do this — Readers

- Drink fluids unless you've been told to restrict.
- Avoid NSAIDs (ibuprofen, naproxen and celecoxib) unless your clinician approves while on certain antibiotics.
- Report reduced urination or swelling promptly.

Do this — Clinicians

- Calculate weight-based dosing and adjust to eGFR; monitor levels when indicated.
- Avoid nephrotoxin stacks; coordinate with pharmacists.
- Set monitoring cadence in the plan (labs, troughs, endpoints).
- Review drug-drug interactions

Conversation starters

- "Do my kidneys need monitoring with this medicine?"
- "Should I avoid ibuprofen while I'm on it?"

Chapter 5
Rhythms of the Heart

"Above all else, guard your heart, for everything you do flows from it."
—Proverbs 4:23

The human heart beats around 100,000 times a day. Each thump feels so ordinary that we hardly notice it, yet its rhythm is the quiet soundtrack of our lives. One stray beat can be enough to change everything. The proverb about guarding the heart speaks not only to emotion but to the fragile cadence of life itself. That rhythm can be thrown into chaos in unexpected ways, even by the very medicines meant to save us.

On a crisp autumn morning in New Mexico, Mario Gonzales woke with a fever and a rattle in his chest. The forty-eight-year-old mechanic and father of two felt a familiar ache—probably bronchitis again, he thought. His doctor prescribed a routine course of azithromycin, the popular "Z-pack" antibiotic, to clear the infection. Mario dutifully picked up the pink pills on his way home. He never imagined that, within days, those pills would nearly snatch his life away.

Two nights later, Mario was lounging on the couch, recovering from his illness and joking with his teenage son, when suddenly he felt his heart lurch. He sat upright. A strange flutter deep in his chest was followed by a rapid, dizzying drumbeat. His vision dimmed at the edges.

"Dad, are you okay?" his son asked, alarmed. Mario opened his mouth to answer, but no words came—a lightning bolt of pain shot through his chest, and he collapsed to the carpet.

At the local emergency department, the cardiac monitors told a frightening story. Mario's heart was galloping erratically, and his blood pressure was plummeting. The electrocardiogram (or ECG) screen showed a jagged, chaotic pattern that his nurses and physician recognized instantly: ventricular tachycardia, a dangerous arrhythmia. In fact, it was devolving into *torsades de pointes* (French for "twisting of the points"), a kind of spiral rhythm that often ends in sudden death. The ER team sprang into action, shouting for the defibrillator. Mario's wife watched from the doorway in horror as his body jolted with the electric shock. After a tense moment, the monitors finally showed a steadier line—the normal sinus rhythm of a heart back from the brink.

Mario survived. Shaken and baffled, he later asked the doctors, "What caused that? I've never had heart problems." When the answer came, Mario's eyes widened in disbelief. The likely culprit was the very antibiotic meant to cure his infection. Azithromycin—a medication millions take every year without a second thought—had sent his heart into deadly fibrillation. How could a simple antibiotic do that?

Mario's case was a wake-up call. In the following days, his doctors pored over medical literature and incident reports. They learned that macrolide antibiotics, the class of drugs including azithromycin, erythromycin, and clarithromycin, have a known, albeit rare, ability to disrupt the heart's electrical rhythm. These antibiotics can prolong the heart's QT interval, an electrical waiting period on the ECG between beats. In some patients, that pause becomes too long—like a stretched rubber band—and the next heartbeat can stumble. If the rhythm degenerates into ventricular fibrillation or torsades de pointes, the result may be sudden cardiac death.

It was not always apparent that these everyday drugs could hold such danger. Erythromycin, one of the oldest macrolides, has been in use since the 1950s. For decades, it was a trusty antibiotic for strep throat and pneumonia. But starting in the 1980s, scattered reports began linking erythromycin to episodes of fainting and deadly arrhythmias. Doctors eventually discovered that erythromycin could block crucial ion channels in the heart and, especially when combined with other medications or in vulnerable patients, trigger cardiac arrest. In one 1990 report, British physicians documented how an intravenous erythromycin infusion led a patient's heart to slip into torsades de pointes– a jarring revelation at the time.

Azithromycin was introduced in the 1990s as a gentler alternative. However, in 2012, a large *New England Journal of Medicine* study shook that assumption. Researchers found that within the first five days of treatment, patients on azithromycin had about 2.5 times the risk of heart-related death compared with those on amoxicillin or no antibiotic. The absolute risk was small, roughly 1 in 20,000, but when a drug is given to millions, rare effects add up.

When people hear that an antibiotic can affect the heart, they picture something dramatic: a pill that can drop you on the floor. That is not what most patients experience. Still, the concern isn't imaginary. A large meta-analysis published in 2015 tried to put a number on the risk and estimated that, across a million courses of treatment, macrolides as a class were associated with about 118 additional ventricular arrhythmias or arrhythmia-related sudden deaths. That sounds scary until you translate it into what it really means: For the vast majority of cases, the absolute risk is still small.

And the story didn't stop there. As newer analyses and better-designed studies came out, the picture became more nuanced and, in many settings, more reassuring. In a large real-world study focused on a high-risk population, researchers found that much of the "extra" cardiac risk reported earlier shrank substantially after adjusting for the types of patients who receive these drugs and the reasons they receive them. Their bottom line was balanced: Most antimicrobials are not linked to a meaningful increase in cardiac events, but azithromycin and clarithromycin may carry a small increased risk in certain situations. The key is not panic, but proportion. When a clinician reaches for a macrolide to treat a serious infection, any modest potential risk has to be weighed against the drug's immediate benefit: Stopping an infection that can harm you far more quickly than a rare arrhythmia.

Some patients face greater danger: the elderly, those with low potassium or magnesium, people with slow resting heart rates, and anyone taking other drugs that affect the heart rhythm. A 2020 study of 4.3 million prescriptions found no extra risk for most patients, but in those already on a QT-prolonging drug, azithromycin raised the odds of fainting or arrhythmia by 40%.

In 2013, the U.S. Food and Drug Administration (FDA) responded to the mounting evidence. They issued a prominent safety warning about azithromycin's potential to cause "potentially fatal irregular heart rhythm," urging caution in patients with existing risk factors. The FDA even updated the antibiotic's label to include warnings about QT prolongation and the rare risk of torsades de pointes. In that same advisory, FDA officials pointed out that azithromycin isn't unique—other macrolides and even fluoroquinolone antibiotics can prolong the QT interval as well. This was a subtle hint of a broader truth: The problem wasn't one rogue drug, but a pattern seen across multiple widely used antibiotics.

Consider clarithromycin, another macrolide often prescribed for respiratory infections. In 2018, the FDA took the unusual step of advising doctors *not to prescribe clarithromycin to patients with heart disease unless no other options were available.* This was based on a long-term clinical trial that found higher rates of heart attacks and deaths among heart patients even years after a short course of clarithromycin. The reasons remain murky—researchers speculated on effects ranging from lingering inflammation to alterations in vascular health—but the message was clear. Regulators around the world, including the European Medicines Agency (EMA), added warnings to clarithromycin's label and urged caution. The World Health Organization (WHO) now flags macrolides as drugs that require careful monitoring because of these rare cardiac side effects and the potential for misuse. After all, more than half of antibiotics worldwide are acquired without a prescription, especially in low- and middle-income countries, meaning millions take these medicines without any professional screening for heart risks.

These antibiotics are household names, used liberally for ear infections, bronchitis, and even acne. They save lives daily by treating serious infections. As one cardiologist noted in a medical journal, "the absolute risk is small, but when a drug is given to millions, even rare harms add up." The challenge is figuring out who is at risk and how to guard those patients while still using these medicines to cure infections.

Global health systems have begun to wrestle with this challenge. In the United States and Europe, guidelines now urge extra caution when prescribing QT-prolonging antibiotics to the elderly or to those with cardiac conditions. Doctors are advised to check for drug interactions, for example, to avoid giving a macrolide to a patient already on an anti-arrhythmic medication or certain diuretics. Hospital pharmacies have implemented alerts: If azithromycin is ordered for a patient on a known QT-prolonging drug, a warning pops up for the physician. These steps are helping in some parts of the world but are not being scaled globally to make a significant impact.

As Mario recovered, halfway across the world another story was unfolding. In a small village clinic in northern India, a grandmother arrived complaining of a severe urinary tract infection. The local doctor faced a dilemma—the clinic had a limited stock of antibiotics, but they did have a powerful drug called ciprofloxacin on hand. Ciprofloxacin is one of the fluoroquinolones, a class of broad-spectrum antibiotics often used for stubborn infections. It's cheap, effective, and widely available—even over-the-counter in some countries.

The doctor administered the drug, grateful to have something potent to treat the infection. The patient recovered from the infection, but a day later, her family reported she had collapsed at home without warning. With no ECG machine or defibrillator in that remote village, no one realized she had suffered the same kind of arrhythmia that struck Mario—likely triggered by the fluoroquinolone meant to heal her.

Fluoroquinolones (often just called "quinolones") include well-known antibiotics like ciprofloxacin (Cipro) and levofloxacin (Levaquin). If you've ever had a tough case of food poisoning or a persistent sinus infection, there's a good chance you've taken one. These drugs are medical workhorses around the globe—used in American outpatient clinics and sub-Saharan African hospitals alike. They have also been under intense scrutiny for safety issues. By the late 1990s and early 2000s, doctors noticed that certain quinolones could cause dangerous heart rhythms, just like the macrolides. In fact, two early drugs in this class—sparfloxacin and gatifloxacin—were pulled from the U.S. and European markets (in 1999 and 2001, respectively) after reports of fatal arrhythmias.

Other fluoroquinolones remained available but with strong warnings on their labels about QT prolongation and rare heart risks.

How considerable is the risk with modern quinolones?

Scientific studies have at times contradicted each other, highlighting how context and patient populations matter. A large Danish-Swedish study in 2016 looked at nearly one million antibiotic treatments and found *no difference* in serious arrhythmia events between people taking fluoroquinolones and those taking penicillin. The most commonly used drug in that study was ciprofloxacin, which may have a relatively lower effect on the heart's electrical cycle. The researchers concluded with a reassuring note: For the average adult, fluoroquinolones did not appear to confer added cardiac risk. This was welcome news, suggesting that these antibiotics could be used without fear for most people, at least when used appropriately.

But other studies have painted a less comforting picture. In Canada, an analysis of health records from the province of Ontario found that certain quinolones were associated with increased odds of sudden death or ventricular arrhythmia, especially in older patients. Moxifloxacin, a potent respiratory quinolone, and levofloxacin were the chief offenders. Back in the United States, a study of veterans (average age fifty-six) revealed that levofloxacin carried significantly higher risks: Over the first ten days of treatment, the risk of serious arrhythmia was elevated in patients on levofloxacin compared with those on amoxicillin. In that same study, azithromycin showed a spike in risk during the first five days, similar to levofloxacin's profile. Notably, when researchers directly compared azithromycin and levofloxacin, they found the two drugs had comparable risks of causing heart rhythm disturbances. The problem of antibiotic-induced arrhythmia spans multiple drug classes.

Digging deeper, cardiologists conducted systematic reviews to make sense of the conflicting data. A 2017 meta-analysis aggregated results from sixteen studies across the globe. The verdict was that fluoroquinolones as a class do modestly increase the risk of serious arrhythmias and even cardiac death. The increase in absolute terms was small—on the order of 160 additional serious arrhythmias per 1,000,000 treatment courses, and 43 additional cardiovascular deaths per 1,000,000 courses. But just as with macrolides, such numbers are not easily dismissed when tens of millions of prescriptions are written each year. The meta-analysis also noted a critical nuance: Not all fluoroquinolones are equal in their impact on the heart. Moxifloxacin and levofloxacin showed the highest risk, whereas ciprofloxacin did not appear to significantly raise arrhythmia risk in the data examined. This aligns with what frontline clinicians suspect—for example, moxifloxacin is known to prolong the QT interval more than ciprofloxacin does. Doctors often avoid moxifloxacin in patients with known heart rhythm issues.

The European Medicines Agency took these findings seriously. By 2018, after reviewing safety data, the EMA imposed stricter regulations on fluoroquinolone use. They highlighted that these drugs should be reserved for cases where there are no other alternative antibiotics, and healthcare professionals should carefully weigh the benefits and risks before prescribing them. Importantly, European regulators sent out safety communications reminding doctors that quinolones can cause not only tendons to rupture and nerves to falter, but also *hearts to misfire.* In practical terms, this means patients with a history of arrhythmia, or those on overlapping medications, should get alternative treatments if possible. Some countries adjusted prescribing guidelines: For instance, in the UK, GPs were urged to avoid prescribing levofloxacin in elderly patients with heart disease.

Call your doctor right away if you feel faint, have a rapid heartbeat, or experience irregular heartbeats. Such warnings aim to do what Proverbs urged long ago: to guard the heart, even at the physical level.

What happens in resource-tight areas?

In low- and middle-income countries, where regulatory oversight can be less stringent, the picture is more complicated. Over-the-counter sales of antibiotics remain common in parts of Asia, Africa, and Latin America. This means a fluoroquinolone might be taken for a simple case of traveler's diarrhea without any medical guidance. In those settings, the safety net of monitoring and warnings is thin. Electrocardiograms are not readily available in many clinics; follow-up is haphazard. If a patient like that Indian grandmother suffers an arrhythmia at home, it may never be officially linked to the antibiotic—the death might be attributed to a "heart attack" or simply go unexamined. Epidemiologists suspect that antibiotic-induced arrhythmias are underreported in developing nations. Global pharmacovigilance data support this concern: The WHO's adverse drug report database (VigiBase) has logged disproportionately more cardiac arrhythmias in patients on fluoroquinolones than in those on other common antibiotics like amoxicillin.

Whether in a bustling U.S. city or a rural village, the underlying biology is the same—these drugs can occasionally derail the heart's electrics—but the outcomes differ drastically depending on resources and awareness.

International health agencies are starting to respond. The WHO has added certain macrolides and fluoroquinolones to its "Watch" category of antibiotics—medicines that are essential but should be used judiciously due to the higher potential for harm and resistance. They have initiated educational campaigns to improve antibiotic use in low-income regions, emphasizing that antibiotics should be respected, not feared: They must be prescribed only when truly necessary and with attention to patient factors that could spell trouble. In some countries, authorities are enacting laws to curb non-prescription sales; for example, India recently moved several antibiotics to a special schedule requiring pharmacists to record purchaser details, an effort to curb unsupervised use. These efforts, while uneven, point toward a growing global recognition of the problem. In essence, the world is relearning an old lesson: Medicines are powerful agents that can heal but also harm if not handled with care.

Back in New Mexico, Mario Gonzales took this lesson to heart—literally. His doctors switched him to a different class of antibiotic to finish treating his bronchitis, one with no effect on heart rhythm. They also scheduled him for a full cardiac workup. Thankfully, Mario's heart itself was fine; it had no underlying disease. An infectious illness, a routine antibiotic, and perhaps a genetic susceptibility had conspired in a perfect storm to pause his wellspring of life. He still gets a lump in his throat when he recalls waking up in the ICU to his wife clutching his hand with tears in her eyes. "It was a miracle," she keeps saying.

Priya's experience

On a hot, windless morning in Chennai, India, Priya Subramanian packed school lunches with one hand and checked lesson plans with the other. She was thirty-eight, a Tamil teacher, a mother of two, and a believer in getting on with things. A week of facial pressure and a blocked nose had slowed her down, so a neighborhood clinic started her on a fluoroquinolone; "strong and fast," the doctor had said. She took the tablets with coffee and went back to her day.

By the fifth morning, the pressure was finally easing. As Priya rinsed steel tiffins and stirred dosa batter, she felt a small flutter in her chest. It was the kind of odd skip you might ignore. Then the flutter became a gallop. Her heart sprinted. The room tilted. A cold, slick sweat gathered at her neck. She called out to her husband and slid to the floor. The ceiling fan blurred into a spinning coin.

The ambulance threaded through auto-rickshaws and buses along Usman Road. In the emergency bay, monitors mapped a storm. Her rhythm was twisting into a dangerous pattern that could collapse without warning. Blood tests ruled out a heart attack. There was no drug use, no thyroid surge, no fever. When the cardiologist realized she had taken cipro-floxacin, the pieces fell into place. A rare reaction had length-ened the heart's electrical reset, tipping her toward torsades de pointes. Years of safety reports had linked certain fluo-roquinolones to this risk. Priya was one of the few unlucky people who felt it.

They stopped the drug and gave her magnesium intrave-nously. The rhythm steadied and the frightening gallop ebbed to a firm, ordinary beat. She stayed overnight in the cardiac unit at a hospital near Mount Road, listening to the soft chorus of monitors and the temple bells drifting in from somewhere beyond the glass. By morning, she could sit up, sip coffee, and take in what had nearly happened.

Back home in West Mambalam, life resumed its familiar cadence: uniforms ironed, violin practice at dusk, a Saturday visit to Marina Beach for corn on the cob. Priya carried a new habit with her. She read the small print on every prescription. She asked about side effects and safer alternatives. She learned that most sinus infections get better on their own, that watchful waiting is often wise, and that when an antibiotic is truly needed, there are gentler first-line choices. "Guard your heart" took on layers of meaning.

Her story is not an indictment of a whole class of medicines. In severe pneumonia or after exposure to dangerous germs, a fluoroquinolone can be lifesaving. In a mild sinus illness, the gamble may not be worth it. That is the quiet lesson Priya repeats to friends over coffee and to parents at school meetings: Every treatment is a balance. Ask what the medicine is for. Ask how long. Ask what could go wrong and what to watch for.

Clinics across India and far beyond are learning the same lesson. Some doctors now ask about palpitations during antibiotic courses. Conferences carve out time for medication safety. Regulators have tightened guidance. Researchers are building better tools to match the right drug to the right patient at the right moment.

As this chapter closes, we return to the proverb that opened it. The heart is strong enough to beat three billion times in a lifetime, yet fragile enough that a tiny molecule can disrupt its rhythm. Respecting that truth is part of practicing wise medicine.

Our next step takes us from the physical to the mental. If an antibiotic can disturb the cadence of the heart, what can it do to the currents of the mind? The next chapter, "Pure Insanity," will take us into stranger territory: stories of antibiotics that have stirred hallucinations, paranoia, even madness. We move from the physical heart to the hidden landscapes of the brain. From guarding your heart… to safeguarding your sanity.

Key ideas

- Some antibiotics prolong the QT interval and can trigger arrhythmias.
- Risk increases with low potassium/magnesium and other QT-prolonging medications.

Do this — Readers

- Share your full med list (including antidepressants, antiemetics, antifungals).
- If you have palpitations, feel faint, or have new dizziness, call.
- Don't start new over-the-counter medications without checking first.

Do this — Clinicians

- Check for QT-drug interactions; correct electrolyte levels; order an ECG if needed.
- Choose non- QT-prolonging alternatives when reasonable.
- Document stop dates and follow-up plans.

Conversation starters

- "Do I take any medications that, combined with this antibiotic, could raise my heart rhythm risk? "
- "Do I need an ECG?"

Chapter 6

Pure Insanity

The Symphony of the Central Nervous System

Imagine the human brain and spinal cord as a grand symphony orchestra. Each neuron is a musician, each region of the nervous system a section of instruments. Together, they perform a seamless concert, conducting every thought, movement, and sensation. When functioning smoothly, this orchestra plays in perfect harmony. The brain's melody governs our heartbeat, the rhythm of our breath, and the clarity of our thoughts. It's an intricate dance that we rarely notice—a quiet, steady background to our lives. But even the most seasoned orchestra can fall into disarray if a single section goes out of tune. A wrong note, a fleeting disruption, can turn an exquisite performance into a cacophony of chaos.

This is the reality for many when medications meant to heal start to unravel the delicate balance within the brain. Select antibiotics can sometimes interfere with the central nervous system in ways no one expects. What begins as a simple treatment can spiral into confusion, hallucinations, and a frightening loss of control. This is a story that spans the world—one that touches patients, families, and healthcare providers alike. It's a tale of misdiagnosis, uncertainty, and the urgent need for awareness of an often-overlooked danger. And at its heart is Grace Fisher, whose life was thrown into turmoil by an antibiotic intended to cure her.

Grace Fisher, a vibrant fifty-six-year-old grandmother, arrived at the hospital with what seemed to be a routine issue: a persistent urinary tract infection. The infection was caused by Pseudomonas aeruginosa, a bacterium well-known for resisting common antibiotics. In response, doctors prescribed cefepime, a potent fourth-generation cephalosporin, typically reserved for more resistant infections. At first, everything seemed to be going according to plan. Her fever from the infection subsided, and Grace began to feel hopeful that her stay in the hospital would be brief.

But as the days passed, subtle changes began to appear. At first, Grace's family chalked it up to the stress of illness. She was a little forgetful, a little groggy—nothing too alarming. But soon, the shift was undeniable. One evening, as her daughter read to her aloud, Grace sat in her hospital bed, staring vacantly past her. Her gaze was distant, almost as if she were seeing something far beyond the room. By midnight, the confusion escalated. Grace began speaking incoherently, plucking at the bedsheets as though she were trying to gather invisible threads. She insisted that strangers were in her room, even though her husband was the only one present. Then, with wide, fearful eyes, Grace whispered about a cat walking on the ceiling, a hallucination that sent a chill down her daughter's spine.

It was a terrifying sight. Grace, once sharp and aware, was drifting in and out of reality, leaving her family helpless and scared. Her daughter clutched her hand, desperate for answers. Was it the infection spreading? Had Grace suffered a stroke? Doctors scrambled to find an explanation. Initially, they suspected ICU delirium, a common type of confusion experienced by critically ill patients. After all, Grace was in the hospital for a serious infection, and she was on strong medication. Specialists were consulted. Tests were run. A CT scan of her brain revealed no abnormalities. Blood work, however, uncovered an important clue: Grace's kidneys were struggling. An acute kidney injury, likely caused by dehydration and the infection, was interfering with her body's ability to clear waste—including medications—from her system.

As her kidneys faltered, the level of cefepime in her bloodstream began to rise. Slowly, almost imperceptibly, the drug that had been intended to help her was building up to toxic levels. And so, in the quiet dark of the hospital room, Grace's mind was slowly being poisoned.

As the night wore on, Grace's condition deteriorated. She became nearly unresponsive, murmuring softly only when the nurses attempted to rouse her. Panic set in. A neurologist was called to investigate. He performed an electroencephalogram, or EEG, to measure the brain's electrical activity. The results were alarming. The EEG showed abnormal slow waves and flickers, signs of toxic encephalopathy—essentially, a brain that had been poisoned and was struggling to function.

It was then that the team made a pivotal decision: stop the cefepime. They switched Grace to a different antibiotic, one less likely to cause harm to her fragile system, and began supportive care. They even considered dialysis, hoping to filter out the toxic drug still circulating in her body.

Slowly, Grace's recovery began. Over the next two days, the fog of confusion lifted. The hallucinations faded away, like the remnants of a bad dream. Her speech became clearer. When she finally recognized her husband and daughter again, there were tears of relief.

Grace had come back from the brink of what seemed like madness, and her family could scarcely believe it.

In the end, it wasn't a stroke or a brain infection that had caused the madness. It wasn't a psychiatric breakdown. It was a commonly prescribed antibiotic, given in good faith, that had caused the damage. Grace's story is far from unique. It's a vivid example of cefepime-induced neurotoxicity, a rare but potentially devastating reaction in which a medication meant to cure throws the brain into chaos. The Fisher family was left stunned, wondering how something so ordinary could go so terribly wrong. Unfortunately, their story is just one of many, a reminder of the fine line between healing and harm when it comes to the powerful drugs we rely on.

How does cefepime affect the brain?

Cefepime, like most antibiotics, is designed to target and kill bacteria. But in some cases, it can unintentionally cause damage to the brain. To understand how, we need to explore the brain's protective barrier and the way cefepime interacts with it.

The brain is shielded by a barrier known as the blood-brain barrier (BBB), which keeps harmful substances from entering. Under normal conditions, cefepime is not meant to cross into the brain in large amounts. But when the drug accumulates in the body, particularly in patients with kidney issues like those that Grace had, it can slip past the BBB. Once inside, cefepime interferes with the brain's chemical signals, specifically targeting GABA receptors. GABA is the brain's braking system, calming excessive neural activity. Cefepime, in effect, disables this brake, allowing the brain's activity to spiral out of control. This disruption can trigger confusion, hallucinations, and agitation—the very symptoms Grace experienced.

Cefepime-induced neurotoxicity, as it's known, can show up in different ways. Early symptoms include confusion, disorientation, and agitation. Some patients may even develop psychosis-like symptoms, such as vivid hallucinations or paranoia. Neurologically, this can also manifest as muscle twitches or tremors, slurred speech, and, in severe cases, seizures. These effects usually appear after a few days of treatment, often when cefepime levels have built up to a critical point in the brain. The good news is that once the drug is stopped, symptoms typically improve within a day or two, with full recovery often within three days.

Who Is at Risk?

While Grace's experience with cefepime-induced neurotoxicity is alarming, it's not as rare as one might think. Studies suggest that about 0.1% to 0.2% of patients on cefepime may experience neurological complications. However, this number rises dramatically in intensive care units (ICUs), where up to 15% of patients on the drug show signs of neurotoxicity.

Certain patients are at higher risk, including the elderly and those with kidney dysfunction. Grace, for example, had an acute kidney injury, which meant her body couldn't clear cefepime efficiently. This allowed the drug to build up in her system, triggering the toxic effects. In fact, impaired kidney function is the most significant risk factor for cefepime neurotoxicity, and improper dosing in patients with kidney issues further increases this risk. Studies have shown that about 80% of patients affected by cefepime neurotoxicity had some degree of kidney dysfunction.

Other factors, like preexisting neurological conditions, high doses, and prolonged use, can also raise the risk. And while most doctors know to adjust the dosage for patients with kidney issues, sometimes the signs of neurotoxicity can be overlooked. Delirium or confusion might be attributed to the illness itself, or other medications, when the real cause is the antibiotic.

Cefepime-induced neurotoxicity is often unrecognized, especially in critical care settings, where symptoms may be dismissed as part of the patient's illness or other treatments. As awareness grows, more cases are being identified, helping to shine a light on this hidden danger. The key takeaway is that although cefepime is a lifesaver for many, it comes with potential risks that shouldn't be overlooked, especially in vulnerable patients. Recognizing and addressing these risks early can make all the difference.

A Global Challenge

Cefepime's neurotoxic effects are well-documented in medical literature, but managing this issue is not just a challenge for one country or hospital; it's a global concern. In high-income countries like the United States and those in Western Europe, awareness and reporting are improving. However, in low- and middle-income countries, where cefepime is widely used, challenges like limited resources and inadequate monitoring can make these side effects harder to detect and manage.

A key issue is the lack of regular kidney function assessments. In many hospitals, especially in resource-limited settings, lab tests may not be done frequently or results may be delayed. Without these tests, doctors may prescribe the standard dosage, even if the patient has undiagnosed kidney problems. This increases the risk of cefepime building up in the body and affecting the brain.

Furthermore, diagnostic tools like EEGs, crucial for detecting subtle brain changes, may be unavailable in poorer regions, leaving cases of neurotoxicity undiagnosed.

Medication safety systems also vary globally. In countries with robust pharmacovigilance systems, adverse reactions like cefepime-induced neurotoxicity are more likely to be reported. But in many places, such reports are rare, meaning the true scope of the issue remains hidden.

Additionally, differences in prescribing practices, such as longer courses or higher doses of cefepime, can increase the risk of toxicity. In resource-poor ICUs, where patients often have multiple risk factors, the ability to adjust treatments and monitor drug levels may be limited. This makes preventing and managing neurotoxicity more challenging. The growing use of cefepime as an affordable generic antibiotic in developing regions may be contributing to an overlooked global problem.

The Wake-Up Call

Cefepime-induced neurotoxicity remained under the radar until 2012, when the FDA issued a warning, emphasizing the importance of dose adjustments for patients with kidney impairment. This alert, along with growing research, brought the issue into focus, leading hospitals to update their protocols and increase awareness. Studies confirmed that even with proper dosing, cefepime could still cause severe neurological side effects, particularly in ICU patients.

Internationally, health agencies began updating guidelines, and by the late 2010s, there was a clearer understanding of how to prevent and manage these toxic effects. Monitoring kidney function, adjusting doses, and watching for neurological changes became standard recommendations. Fortunately, most patients recover fully once the drug is stopped, but only if the neurotoxicity is recognized in time.

While the 2012 FDA alert was a critical moment, the journey to better antibiotic safety is ongoing. Cefepime is just one example of how potent antibiotics can have unexpected effects on the brain. As awareness grows, it serves as a reminder that prescribing antibiotics requires balancing benefits with risks, a lesson learned from cases like Grace's.

Fluoroquinolone Nightmares

Cefepime is not the only antibiotic that can unsettle the brain. Fluoroquinolones, a family of drugs prescribed every day for routine problems like sinusitis and bronchitis, can cause similar problems. For most people, they work. For some, they spark a different kind of storm. Patients describe sleepless nights, racing thoughts, sudden panic, and even vivid hallucinations. The same orchestra of the nervous system can lose its rhythm, this time from pills that sit in many home medicine cabinets.

How does this happen? Fluoroquinolones can enter the brain and irritate the very circuits that keep activity balanced. Like cefepime, they can blunt the calming effect of GABA, the brain's natural brake, which helps explain insomnia, agitation, and paranoia. They can also injure peripheral nerves, the long, delicate cables that carry sensation from skin and muscle to the spinal cord. Research suggests these drugs may stress nerve cells' energy factories and trigger inflammation, leaving fibers hypersensitive or numb. The result is a double hit: the mind on edge, the body buzzing or burning.

Burning Feet

On a warm April night in Phoenix, when the desert air still holds the day's heat, Calvin slid into bed and noticed a strange fizzing in his feet. He was forty-five, a weekend runner who liked the sunrise loop on South Mountain and Saturday hikes on the Mogollon Rim when the family could get away. He had started ciprofloxacin a few days earlier for a routine sinus infection. By midweek, the tingling spread. Pins and needles turned into hot wires. He fumbled with shirt buttons. The tile floor felt like shifting gravel, as if his toes had forgotten how to read it.

His primary care doctor checked for the usual suspects: Diabetes. Thyroid disease. Vitamin levels. All normal. A neurologist tapped a reflex hammer and asked a plain question. Any new medicines? When Calvin said "ciprofloxacin," the room went quiet. The timing lined up with a pattern that clinicians know, and many patients learn the hard way. Fluoroquinolone-induced peripheral neuropathy can start within days. It can feel like burning, electric shocks, numbness, or a loss of fine touch that makes a flat floor feel unsteady.

They stopped the antibiotic at once. The sinus symptoms had already faded. The nerve symptoms did not. Not at first. Pain management helped him sleep. Physical therapy taught him to steady his gait and protect his numb toes from blistering on hot pavement. Little by little, some sensation crept back. The easy sunrise run never fully returned. He learned to plan around the heat and the footing. Family hikes in Sedona became shorter out-and-back trails with water breaks in the shade of cottonwoods. He graded progress in small wins. A mailbox walk without the shock of hot stone underfoot. A morning on the greenbelt with his kids without needing to sit down.

Most people do well on fluoroquinolones. Many never feel more than a queasy stomach. A meaningful minority do not, and the harm can be serious and slow to unwind. That truth has pushed regulators and clinicians to adjust how these medicines are used. Shorter courses. Narrower indications. A careful pause before choosing them for routine infections when safer options exist.

Arizona families will recognize the practical lessons in Calvin's story. Footing matters when sidewalks heat like griddles by noon. Hydration matters when the thermometer climbs past 100°F. Nerves that misfire turn ordinary ground into a challenge. The larger lesson reaches beyond one state. The central nervous system is a delicate stage. When a treatment begins to play the wrong tune, we have to hear it quickly and change the music.

Mark's Plight: When the Cure Feels Like the Disease

On a sticky July afternoon in Atlanta, Mark noticed a painful boil on his thigh. He was thirty-two, an engineer and newlywed who split his time between Midtown job sites and late dinners along Peachtree. Urgent care drained the boil and sent him home with trimethoprim–sulfamethoxazole, the familiar Bactrim, so he could get back to work before Monday.

For a few days, the plan seemed to work. The redness shrank and the soreness faded. Then, one week later, a new problem arrived, like a thunderstorm over the Downtown Connector. Mark woke with a splitting headache, a fever that climbed fast, and a neck that refused to bend. Even the lamp on the nightstand felt like a blade of light. His wife drove him to the emergency department, where the calm of the emergency room turned into a rush of IV drips, a spinal tap, and medical scans.

The spinal fluid was clear. No bacteria grew on the cultures. Yet everything about Mark looked like meningitis. His blood pressure drifted, the fever spiked again, and for a few hours, he struggled to follow simple questions. An infectious diseases specialist joined the team and walked the timeline back. The turn had come after starting Bactrim. A rare possibility rose to the top of the list: drug-induced aseptic meningitis.

They stopped the antibiotic and watched closely. Within twenty-four hours, his fever softened. By forty-eight hours, the headache had retreated to a dull echo, and his neck loosened. He went home tired, sore, and rattled, carrying the uneasy truth that a routine antibiotic had nearly impersonated one of the most feared infections.

Bactrim's effect on the brain differs from what we see with fluoroquinolones or cefepime. In a small number of people, the immune system misreads the drug as a threat and inflames the meninges, the thin membranes around the brain and spinal cord. The spinal fluid shows inflammation without microbes, which is why symptoms can look severe while cultures stay negative. You stop the drug, and the storm usually passes, although the memory of it can linger.

Back in their apartment near Piedmont Park, Mark and his wife made a new habit. Every clinic visit began with a careful list of medicines. He learned to speak up early if a headache felt different, and to ask about alternatives when antibiotics were suggested for skin infections. The boil healed. Life in Atlanta returned to its familiar rhythms, only now with a little more caution, and a lot more respect for antibiotics.

From Anxiety to Psychosis: What Patients Report

Across countries and ages, people have described a similar arc after starting fluoroquinolones. Rising anxiety. Sleepless nights. Confusion. In some, vivid hallucinations or crushing depression. Older adults tend to show delirium or psychosis. Younger adults more often report panic, agitation, or dark mood swings. Many have no psychiatric history. A few cases have ended in tragedy, which pushed regulators to act.

By 2016, the United States added a black box warning to all fluoroquinolones for serious neurological and psychiatric risks, alongside tendon and nerve warnings. Labels now tell clinicians to avoid these drugs for minor infections and to stop therapy at the first sign of mental status change. Europe followed with strict limitations in 2019, urging the use only when safer options do not work. The United Kingdom strengthened warnings again in 2023, including alerts about suicidal thoughts. These steps do not ban the drugs; they ask for care and precision.

Who Is Most at Risk?

Anyone can be affected, but some groups are more vulnerable.

Older adults clear drugs more slowly and often take multiple medications. The same dose that causes mild insomnia in a young person can tip a senior into delirium. Critically ill patients walk a narrow ledge. Infection, inflammation, and sedatives strain the brain. Add a fluoroquinolone, and the balance can fail. In these settings, what looks like "ICU psychosis" may be a medication effect.

In many low- and middle-income regions, antibiotics can be purchased without close supervision. Fluoroquinolones and Bactrim are common, cheap, and often taken without guidance about risks or interactions.

A farmer who develops burning feet after a course of pills may never hear the word neuropathy. A grandmother who becomes confused on therapy may be labeled as having dementia. Limited diagnostics and underreporting hide the real burden.

What to Watch For, What to Do?

Timing matters. New agitation, insomnia, confusion, visual or tactile hallucinations, electric or burning pain in the limbs, or sudden severe headache and fever that begin days after starting an antibiotic should raise suspicion. Tell the prescriber. Do not take additional doses while the cause is being assessed. Clinicians should consider drug interactions, kidney function, and the availability of safer alternatives. When the offending drug is stopped early, the brain and nerves often recover. If symptoms are severe, hospital care, EEG, and supportive treatment may be needed.

The Lasting Toll: Lives Altered in Silence

What do these side effects look like in real life? For Calvin, they meant the end of marathons and the start of a daily negotiation with burning nerves. For Mark, they meant a night in the ER that felt like the edge of death, then weeks of lost income and the echo of fear every time a headache arrived. Multiply their stories by thousands, and you will begin to see a quiet epidemic. These injuries rarely announce themselves. There is no cast or scar. A coworker sees a limp and assumes a sprain. A friend hears "hospital" and thinks the infection was the villain. The medication is invisible, so the harm feels invisible, too.

That invisibility strains trust. Patients who connect their symptoms to a recent antibiotic are sometimes dismissed. "It's all in your head," one doctor said to a woman who developed panic and depression after levofloxacin. It was in her head, just not in the way he meant.

The emotional fallout can be heavy. People describe a sense of betrayal, a grief for the body they had before the pills. Some find community online and learn practical ways to cope. Others sink under the weight of pain or relentless anxiety. A few, in the darkest moments, consider ending their lives. Each of those losses is a tragedy, especially when the original illness was routine.

Clinicians are learning to hold two truths at once. Antibiotics save lives. In a small but significant minority, they also cause life-altering harm. Every prescription becomes a balancing act. Is the drug truly needed, at this dose, for this duration, in this patient? Conversations about risk are becoming part of informed consent, empowering but also unsettling. With hindsight, Calvin likely could have received a safer option for sinusitis. Mark's history hinted at sulfa sensitivity, a clue that might have steered his medical team elsewhere. Each story points to the same goal: better guidance, earlier recognition, fewer injuries.

High Stakes and Quiet Tragedies: A Glimpse Ahead

As Calvin rebuilt his routines and Mark regained strength, both men realized how close they had come to medicine's unintended edge. They started to ask a harder question. How many others are out there with stories that ended worse? A sister's sudden seizure on levofloxacin. A neighbor's unexplained fall after new numbness in the feet. A suicide that followed a cascade of insomnia and panic during treatment. These are the cases that rarely make it into charts as drug reactions. They are filed under stroke, or accident, or depression, with no mention of the recent prescription.

The lesson is not to fear antibiotics. It is to respect them. Use the right drug, at the right dose, for the right time, with eyes open to warning signs. Stop early if the mind or nerves begin to falter. Offer patients clear information and a plan for what to do if something feels off. Build systems that flag risk and invite second looks. And when in doubt, consult an infectious diseases specialist for help.

As this chapter closes, we carry what Calvin and Mark taught us. Medicine is powerful and imperfect. The victories are real, and so are the costs. In the next chapter, "Excess Deaths," we will follow the evidence and the stories that suggest some losses have gone unnoticed, hidden in plain sight. The questions are hard. How do we account for lives quietly lost? How do we balance lifesaving care with life-altering risk? And how do we make sure that the tools we use to heal do not become the source of harm? The answers begin with our willingness to learn and change.

Key ideas
- Certain antibiotics can cause insomnia, agitation, hallucinations, or seizures—especially in older adults or those with renal impairment.
- Early recognition and prompt switch are imperative.

Do this — Readers
- Tell someone you trust you're starting a new antibiotic; ask them to watch for cognitive and mood changes.
- If you develop new confusion, agitation, or severe insomnia, contact your team.
- Avoid driving if you feel mentally "off."

Do this — Clinicians
- Screen for prior neuro events; dose-adjust in CKD; caution in elders.

- Provide explicit return precautions for neuropsychiatric symptoms.
- Switch class promptly if effects appear.

Conversation starters

- "Could this medicine affect my sleep or thinking?"
- "When should I stop and call you?"

For the everyday side effects that push people to quit early or self-treat, see the Bonus Chapter: "Small Harms, Big Consequences." You can also visit *beyondthecurebook.com*

Chapter 7
Excess Death

Alpen Patel was a grandfather of four. One crisp autumn evening, he arrived in the emergency department, feverish, confused, and gasping for air. The team suspected sepsis, a body-wide infection that can turn fatal in hours, and they moved fast. Following protocol, they started vancomycin and piperacillin-tazobactam. Zosyn, as it is known on the wards, is the hospital workhorse when the source is unclear. It casts a wide net. His family took comfort in that. The "big guns" were on board.

In the ICU, Alpen's numbers wavered. At first, the fever eased, and hope returned. Then his kidneys faltered, his blood pressure dipped, and a slow cascade began. Despite careful care, organ after organ struggled. When Alpen died, those in the room felt stunned.

Everyone had done the right things, or so it seemed. How could a best-practice choice end this way?

A clue emerged from research that compared two common combinations for suspected sepsis. Patients who received vancomycin with piperacillin-tazobactam did worse, on average, than those who received vancomycin with cefepime. The difference was small for any single person, but real at the population level. One extra death for roughly every twenty patients treated with the broader regimen. Multiply that across hospitals and years, and the quiet toll grows large.

Why would two effective treatments diverge? The answer may lie in the gut. Our intestines house dense communities of bacteria that help digest food, train the immune system, and crowd out troublemakers. Piperacillin-tazobactam does not just hit the invader; it sweeps up many of these guardians, especially anaerobes that thrive without oxygen. When those communities are erased, the gut barrier may become leaky, inflammation may smolder, and fragile organs may tip from recovery to failure even after the infection is controlled.

Think of a garden stripped of groundcover. Rain comes, soil washes away, and weeds take over an area where protection once stood.

The most persuasive evidence came from a natural experiment. During a nationwide shortage of piperacillin-tazobactam, hospitals switched to cefepime by necessity.

Outcomes improved. Patients had more days free of organ failure and were less likely to die in the months after sepsis. Nothing exotic changed at the bedside, only the choice of which IV bag to hang.

For decades, the mantra in sepsis has been simple. Cover everything, and do it quickly. That instinct saves lives when the clock is ticking. Yet Alpen's story, and the data that followed, suggest there is a cost to blanket coverage. When we carpet-bomb the microbiome, we sometimes hurt the patient we are trying to save.

This is not an argument against urgency. It is a call for precision. Start fast, but start wisely. If broad anaerobic coverage is not clearly needed, reach for narrower options and reassess daily. De-escalate the antibiotics as soon as cultures, imaging, and clinical course allow. The smallest choices, made in the first hour, can ripple for months. In Alpen's case, no one could have known in the moment that a different combination might have given him a better chance. Now that we do, our responsibility is to let that knowledge shape the next patient with sepsis, and the one after that.

Unseen Killers

Alpen's story was not an outlier. Many antibiotics, used without careful thought, can cause harm that has nothing to do with resistance or classic allergies. The trouble often unfolds quietly, in the background, while everyone focuses on the infection.

Consider Barbara, an older woman living well with heart disease. She took an ACE inhibitor (lisinopril) for blood pressure and a small daily spironolactone to help her heart and conserve potassium. When she developed a urinary infection, her doctor prescribed trimethoprim–sulfamethoxazole, the familiar Bactrim. A week later, her son found her collapsed. In the hospital, her potassium was dangerously high, a condition called hyperkalemia. Too much potassium scrambles the heart's electrical signals, like overloading a battery. Trimethoprim can make the kidneys hold on to potassium, and in someone already on potassium-raising medicines, that extra nudge can trigger a fatal rhythm. Extensive studies show this combination raises the risk of hospitalization and sudden death when compared with safer choices like amoxicillin. The warning signs are subtle. There is no rash or wheeze, only a collapse that looks like "heart trouble. "

Another example is metronidazole, a trusty antibiotic discovered in the 1950s and commonly used for gut infections or deep dental abscesses. It's superb at wiping out anaerobic bacteria and is a go-to treatment for serious gut infections like *Clostridioides difficile* colitis and certain parasitic diseases. But if you give metronidazole to someone who might not truly need such broad anaerobic coverage, you could be wreaking havoc on their gut microbiome for little to no benefit. Research has shown that metronidazole can drastically alter the intestinal microbial balance. Patients who receive this drug for diarrhea sometimes don't recover any faster than those who go without it. However, they often end up with a profoundly altered gut flora that can take a long time to return to normal. Some individuals even report lingering digestive troubles and a sense that their stomach never quite "felt right" after a course of metronidazole. While metronidazole's immediate side effects (like nausea or that infamous metallic taste in the mouth) are well known, these subtle, longer-term effects on the body's natural microbial community are only beginning to be understood. Such changes might not directly kill a patient, but they could set the stage for future health issues or vulnerabilities.

The Most Vulnerable at Greatest Risk

Those with fragile organs carry the heaviest burden. In patients with reduced kidney function, the pairing of vancomycin with piperacillin–tazobactam drives up the risk of acute kidney injury when compared with vancomycin plus cefepime. Once the kidneys stumble, fluids accumulate, toxins rise, and other drugs are not cleared. An ICU course that looked stable on day two can unravel by day five, with fluid in the lungs and falling blood pressure. The infection appears controlled, yet the patient declines. Often, the first domino was renal stress made worse by our antibiotic choice.

Polypharmacy, defined as taking five or more simultaneous prescriptions, adds more tripwires. An older adult on medicines for heart failure, diabetes, and arthritis walks a narrow ridge. Add Bactrim and potassium can spike. Add metronidazole or Bactrim to warfarin (a commonly prescribed anticoagulant to prevent blood clots in high-risk individuals), and bleeding risk jumps because these antibiotics slow warfarin's breakdown. The result can be an emergency visit for internal bleeding that no one immediately links to last week's prescription.

The lesson is not to fear antibiotics; it is to respect them. Ask what the infection is most likely to be, choose the narrowest agent that will work, and check the medication list for interactions. In patients with kidney or heart disease, plan for labs and follow-up. If there is no apparent need for broad anaerobic coverage, spare the microbiome. Every prescription sends ripples through a person's biology. For those already standing in deep water, even small waves can pull them under.

Rethinking Antibiotics: Individualized Care and Conversation

The lesson from Alpen and Barbara is simple. Power helps, precision heals. The goal is not bigger coverage, it is a better match between the drug and the person.

At the bedside, that begins with the patient in front of us. What is the likely source of infection? What organs are already fragile? Which medicines are on the home list? If the source of the sepsis doesn't look to be coming from the abdomen, vancomycin with cefepime may be safer than adding anaerobic coverage that the gut does not need. If an older patient on an ACE inhibitor and spironolactone needs treatment for a urinary infection, choose a safer option than Bactrim or, at a minimum, check potassium within a few days. Narrow early when culture data arrive. Reassess daily. Small choices in the first hour can change the patient's life in month three.

Conversation is part of the prescription. Patients deserve to know not only what to take, but why this drug, what to watch for, and when to call. Instead of a quick warning about nausea or rash, add a plan. "Because you are on a blood pressure pill that can raise potassium, we will check labs in five days." Clear expectations turn vague unease into concrete safety steps. They also soften the common belief that stronger is always better.

Sometimes the right antibiotic is the one that treats today's germ while leaving tomorrow's body intact.

Hospitals are building these habits into protocols. Stewardship teams nudge clinicians toward the right drug, dose, and duration, and away from unnecessary anaerobic coverage. The same shift is happening globally. Guidelines are being updated, and training now emphasizes matching the medicine to the person, not to the widest imaginable microbe list.

None of this makes antibiotics villains. They remain among the greatest gifts of modern medicine. The point is to use them with intention and be cognizant of collateral effects.

Paul's story shows why that matters. He was sixty-eight, a retired teacher, steady with his health. A winter cough earned him clarithromycin, a common antibiotic. He added the pills to his pillbox beside his daily diltiazem, a calcium channel blocker for blood pressure.

Within days of taking these two together, he grew dizzy and pale. One morning, he collapsed. In the emergency department, his pressure was dangerously low, and his kidneys were faltering.

The culprit was the combination. Clarithromycin can block the liver pathway that clears diltiazem. With clearance slowed, diltiazem levels rise, blood vessels relax too much, pressure falls, and organs are starved of blood. No new disease, just two routine medicines working against each other. Paul recovered, shaken but wiser. A different antibiotic would likely have avoided the crisis. He almost lost his life.

This is individualized care in practice. Before prescribing, scan the med list for known clashes. Ask about kidney and heart disease. Choose the narrowest effective drug. Tell patients what abnormal symptoms matter, and arrange the lab checks that can catch trouble early. The result is quiet safety, fewer spirals into kidney failure after broad coverage, fewer sudden arrhythmias from hidden potassium spikes, and fewer collapses like Paul's.

The stories above flow into a single aim. Treat the infection, protect the person. Use the right drug, for the right bug, in the right person with a plan. When we pair precision with conversation, lifesaving medicines do more saving and far less harm.

When Medicines Collide: A Hidden Danger

Paul's crisis was not a fluke; it was a textbook drug interaction hiding in plain sight. Picture the liver as a busy factory where enzymes break down medicines. Clarithromycin slows a key enzyme, CYP3A4. Diltiazem, Paul's blood pressure pill, relies on that enzyme to be cleared at a steady pace. With the pathway blocked, diltiazem accumulated day by day until his vessels relaxed too much, his pressure collapsed, and his kidneys were starved of blood. Neither drug is unsafe by itself. Together, in the wrong pairing, they can become dangerous. This is the peril that lives between prescriptions, a cough treated here and hypertension managed there, without checking how the medicines share the same route through the liver. The fallout shows up as dizziness, a faint on the bathroom floor, a sudden ICU admission, even death—all of it preventable.

The evidence has been clear for years. Extensive studies in older adults show that combining macrolide antibiotics such as clarithromycin or erythromycin with calcium channel blockers sharply increases the risk of severe hypotension, kidney injury, and death. The pattern is specific. Azithromycin, which does not block CYP3A4, does not carry the same danger. Some blood pressure medicines are riskier than others, but most that rely on CYP3A4 can be affected.

The fix is simple in principle. Choose a non-interacting antibiotic when possible, or adjust the blood pressure drug and watch closely. Do a quick medication review, explain what to watch for, and arrange the lab checks that catch trouble early.

Avoidable Harm, Ordinary Fixes

The hardest part of Paul's story is how preventable it was. A different antibiotic, azithromycin, would likely have spared him the collapse. A pharmacy alert could have triggered a quick phone call and a changed prescription. The hypotension and kidney injury were not fate, they were the product of a pairing we already know to avoid. Researchers have estimated that in a single region, hundreds of hospitalizations and deaths trace back to this combination. Each number is a person, a family, a crisis that did not have to happen.

Regulators warned us. The FDA flagged the risk of severe low blood pressure when clarithromycin is taken with calcium channel blockers metabolized by CYP3A4, including verapamil, amlodipine, and diltiazem. Yet the message often stalled before it reached the clinic. Modern care is crowded. Doctors race through full schedules, patients arrive with long medication lists, and no one can hold every interaction in mind. Familiar habits add friction. If clarithromycin has seemed safe for years, warnings can feel abstract.

Communication gaps widen the risk. A cardiologist assumes the primary care doctor will remember the interaction. The primary care doctor trusts the pharmacist's software to catch it. The pharmacist assumes the prescriber has weighed the tradeoffs. Everyone is responsible, so no one is. Patients, unwarned, swallow a hidden hazard.

The result is a blind spot that only becomes visible in the emergency department or the obituary. Each case is a missed chance to choose a non-interacting antibiotic, adjust the blood pressure medicine, or arrange a brief check of blood pressure and kidney function. The fixes are simple, but they require attention.

There is movement in the right direction. Electronic health records now fire bright warnings when risky pairs are ordered. Paul tells his friends to bring an updated medication list and to ask pharmacists about interactions. Still, avoidable drug collisions remain common. In an age of medical miracles, one of our most reliable safety tools is ordinary vigilance, shared by clinicians, pharmacists, and patients who ask the small questions that prevent the significant harms.

A Global Problem, Hiding in Plain Sight

It is tempting to file Paul's story under local practice, a North American quirk. It is not. The world is full of antibiotics and blood pressure pills, which means the potential for dangerous combinations exists everywhere. Macrolides like clarithromycin are among the most used antibiotics on the planet. At the same time, hypertension is now universal, and calcium channel blockers such as amlodipine and diltiazem sit on medicine shelves from city pharmacies to rural clinics.

Put those facts together, and the overlap is inevitable. Millions of people who take a daily blood pressure pill will, at some point, be given an antibiotic for a cough, a sinus infection, or pneumonia. In many countries, antibiotics can be bought without a doctor's visit, records are scattered, and prescribers may never see the full medication list. The risk is not theoretical. It is built into the way care is delivered.

Infrastructure shapes outcomes. Paul had paramedics at his door within minutes and an emergency department that could piece together the puzzle. In a remote village or an overcrowded city hospital, the same collapse can be misread as a stroke or a heart attack. The pharmacy label is thrown away, the interaction is never named, and the death is folded into statistics that say nothing about cause.

These are excess deaths that pass quietly, multiplied by distance and limited resources.

Even in well-resourced systems, the hazard persists. Europe's aging population relies on both antibiotics and calcium channel blockers. Electronic alerts help, but busy clinics override warnings, or the recommended drug for a penicillin allergy happens to be clarithromycin. A small gap in communication, a rushed decision, and a familiar pairing slip through.

This is what public health calls a silent epidemic. There is no outbreak to map, no rash to photograph, only scattered emergencies that look unrelated until you zoom out. The pattern repeats across borders. The same drug pair. The same dizziness and collapse. The same preventable harm.

Recognizing the scale is the first step. The solutions are not exotic. Teach clinicians to scan for collisions, favor non-interacting antibiotics when possible, and build pharmacy systems that flag high-risk pairs clearly. Strengthen prescription oversight where antibiotics are sold freely. Offer simple guidance for patients on long-term heart or kidney medicines, so they know to ask before starting a new antibiotic. Small steps, repeated everywhere, can turn this quiet problem into a visible one, and visibility is how we begin to fix it.

And it's not only drug pairs that collide. Sometimes the collision is between an antibiotic and the body's most fragile balances.

Two Quiet Metabolic Traps

Blood sugar swings: when the numbers drift, then swing
Not all antibiotic harm announces itself with a rash or a new pain. Sometimes it shows up as a number that drifts, then swings.

If you're older, or you live with diabetes, a new antibiotic can nudge blood sugar in the wrong direction. Sometimes it climbs and won't come down. Sometimes it drops fast and feels frightening: sweating, shaking, confusion, sudden weakness, a strange sense that you can't think straight. The danger isn't only the glucose. It's what comes next. A fall in the bathroom. A near-miss on the road. Delirium that looks like "just being tired." A bad night that turns into an ambulance ride.

That's why this matters. Not because blood sugar swings always kill, but because they can be the first domino in someone who doesn't have much reserve.

Practical protection: If you have diabetes, or you care for someone who does, treat the first week of a new antibiotic as a week to pay closer attention. Check sugars a little more often. Keep quick sugar nearby. And if someone suddenly "acts different" after starting an antibiotic, don't assume it's only the infection or age. Check a fingerstick and call.

Hyperkalemia: the slow rise that can end abruptly
Potassium is one of those lab values that feels invisible until it isn't. When potassium rises, the heart can become electrically unstable. Sometimes there are no early clues. Sometimes the clues are easy to dismiss: unusual weakness, heaviness

in the limbs, nausea, or a fatigue that doesn't match the day. In higher-risk people, the first clear sign can be palpitations, dizziness, or a rhythm problem that comes out of nowhere.

The people most vulnerable are often the ones already juggling several risks: chronic kidney disease, dehydration, diabetes, and medications that tend to raise potassium. Many patients know these medications by nickname, not category: "my blood pressure pill," "my water pill," "the one for my heart."

Add a risky antibiotic to that stack, and the safety margin shrinks.

Practical protection: If you've ever been told your kidneys are "not great," or you take medicines for blood pressure, heart failure, or kidney issues, ask one simple question when an antibiotic is prescribed: "Do I need a potassium check?" And if you develop new weakness, a heavy, washed-out feeling, faintness, or palpitations after starting an antibiotic, call. This is one of those problems where catching it early can change the ending."Sometimes it's a drug pair.

Sometimes it's a lab value. Either way, the end of the story can look the same." And when it does, it rarely feels like a side effect. It feels like fate.

The Human Cost of Overlooking the Details

Behind every percentage point is a person. For Paul Lanzoni, the number became a night of fear, a sudden drop from a routine cough to failing organs. For his wife, it was the shock of finding him on the floor and the dread that a simple antibiotic might make her a widow.

Others never get answers. An elderly woman dies quietly at home, and it is called natural causes. A man with heart disease is found unresponsive, and the blame falls on his heart, not on the ordinary pills that collided in his bloodstream.

These are excess deaths, injuries beyond what the illness alone would have caused, and harms attributable to the treatments meant to help. It is a bitter paradox. In trying to cure the cough, the system nearly killed the patient by amplifying another condition. The pattern persists because care often happens in silos. One clinician treats the infection. Another manages the blood pressure. The left hand assumes the right will catch the details. In those gaps, people fall.

The toll is not only physical. There is pain from kidney injury, the terror of a collapse, the fog of an ICU stay. There is anger and a sense of betrayal, a crack in trust. How do you tell a family that the threat came from the medicine meant to cure and not from the disease?

Clinicians feel it, too. Many carry the memory of a case that went wrong because of something they ordered, despite their best intentions. Systems and safeguards exist, yet holes remain.

Much of the damage is invisible. For every hospitalization we count, there may be dozens of near misses, a faint that does not become a fall, a kidney strain that never reaches a lab result, a death filed under another cause. It is an iceberg problem, a small tip we can see and a larger mass below the waterline. Grief deepens when families realize a loss might have been avoidable. If only the interaction had been flagged. If only a different antibiotic had been chosen. If only someone had said, "Let's check your labs in a few days." Those questions haunt the people who loved the patient and the clinicians who cared for them. Every prescription deserves a brief pause to check for interactions, a clear explanation of warning signs, and a plan to follow up. That is how trust is rebuilt, one careful decision at a time.

Looking Ahead: A Slow Poison Brewing

As Paul regained his strength, a more complex question emerged. If a week of antibiotics can push a healthy man to the edge, what happens when medicines are taken for months or years? Not the thunderclap, but the slow leak. Subtle shifts in the body's balance, quiet strain on organs, a microbiome reshaped until the consequences surface far downstream.

That is where we go next. In "Slow Poison: The Cost of Long-Term Use," we follow patients whose warnings were not dramatic, only persistent. We will map the small changes that accumulate, the risks that grow with time, and the choices that can prevent them. The goal is not blame. It is light. With each story, we learn how to keep powerful tools from becoming hidden harms, and how to bring more people like Alpen Patel safely home.

Key ideas
- Overuse and inappropriate choices can worsen outcomes at the population level.
- Matching drug, dose, and duration to true need saves lives.

Do this — Readers
- Ask what bacteria we're targeting and how we'll know it's working.
- Keep vaccines up to date and use infection-prevention habits (hand hygiene).
- Never share leftover antibiotics or keep "just in case."
- Always carry an updated list of your medications with you

Do this — Clinicians

- Indication + duration on every order; decide in forty-eight to seventy-two hours if you need to continue antibiotics
- Track local resistance; align with guidelines and formulary stewardship.
- De-escalate or stop when cultures/clinical course allow.
- Check for drug-drug interactions and weigh benefits vs risks. Consider alternatives. First-line agents are not first-line for everyone.

Conversation starters

- "How will we reassess this antibiotic in forty-eight to seventy-two hours?"
- "What signs mean we can stop sooner?"
- "How will my other medications affect this antibiotic?"

Chapter 8

Slow Poison: The Cost of Long-Term Use

Sarah Vandyk never imagined an ordinary antibiotic could steal her breath. In her mid-forties, healthy and active, she dealt with a nuisance that many women know well: recurring urinary tract infections. Her doctor prescribed nitrofurantoin, a small brown pill that has been around since the 1950s. It can end a urinary tract infection fast, and for people with frequent infections, some take it every day to prevent the next one. Sarah did exactly that. For months, the plan worked. No burning, no late-night clinic visits, just relief.

Then the stairs to her apartment felt steeper. Cold mornings brought a dry cough that would not leave. She told herself it was the tail end of a virus, or maybe stress. Weeks passed. Bringing groceries in from the car, her chest tightened, and the world tilted. She sat on the curb, gulping air as if through a straw.

At the clinic, her doctor heard faint crackles deep in her lungs. An X-ray showed hazy new shadows. Pneumonia was the first guess. Heart trouble was another. A lung specialist asked a different question. "What medicines have you been taking for a long time?" Sarah listed only one: nitrofurantoin. The room went quiet.

Further tests gave the answer. Her lung tissue was stiffening and scarring, a process called pulmonary fibrosis. In rare cases, nitrofurantoin can set off the immune system in a way that injures the lungs. Sometimes the reaction is sudden, like an allergic storm.

Sometimes it is slow, a quiet injury that builds month by month until breathing feels tight all the time. Most people take this medicine without anything more than nausea or a headache. A small number experience serious harm. Sarah had become one of them.

She stopped the drug that day. Stopping early matters. For some, the lungs calm down and the abnormal CT scans clear over time. For Sarah, the free fall ended, and the cough eased, but the scars did not vanish. Weekend hikes turned into careful walks with the dog. She learned to pace her breaths and listen to her body in a way she never had before.

What happened to Sarah is uncommon, yet it teaches a simple truth. Medicines have two stories. The first is the help they give. The second is what can happen when they are used longer than needed or without a plan to check for trouble. Nitrofurantoin is a good antibiotic for short hits. Taken daily for months, especially without lung check-ins, it can, rarely, become a slow poison.

There are safer ways to use it. Treat the infection, then stop. If prevention is truly needed, set a time limit and a follow-up. Ask about new cough, chest tightness, or breathlessness, even if it seems minor. A quick pause to rethink the plan can protect the lungs that carry us through our days.

Sitting by her window at dusk, Sarah traced the outlines of a life adjusted but not ended. She was grateful to know the cause, even if the knowledge arrived late. Each breath was a reminder that small pills are powerful, and that the safest medicine is the one taken with care, a clear goal, and a finish line. Sarah was not alone. Thousands of miles away, Bruce Lou learned that an antibiotic could injure a very different part of the body.

Bruce was fifty-two, fit, and proud of it. An intestinal infection earned him a prescription for ciprofloxacin. The pills worked; his fever and diarrhea resolved. A week after finishing the antibiotic, he laced up for a morning jog and, while running, he felt a sharp pop in his heel, then fire. He crumpled to the pavement. His Achilles tendon had snapped.

At the hospital, an orthopedic surgeon asked a simple question. "Any recent medications?" When Bruce said "ciprofloxacin," the surgeon nodded. Fluoroquinolone antibiotics can rarely inflame or weaken tendons, including the Achilles. The risk is higher with age or steroid use, but it can happen to younger people, too. Scientists think these drugs may damage collagen, the scaffolding that gives tendons strength. The United States placed a strong warning on these medicines years ago for exactly this reason. Most people never have a problem. A few do, and the injury can be life-changing.

Bruce spent weeks in a cast, then months relearning how to walk without a limp. He was grateful to heal, yet angry that no one had warned him to go easy on his legs after the prescription. A short course for a stomach bug had stolen his stride for an entire season.

Around the same time, Abdul Karim, sixty-four, finished a two-week course of ciprofloxacin for a stubborn urinary infection. Two weeks later, a stabbing pain ripped across his chest and back. In the emergency department, scans showed a tear in his aorta, the largest artery in the body. Surgeons raced the clock and saved his life.

Only afterward did a doctor connect the dots. Research suggests that fluoroquinolones can, in rare cases, make the walls of arteries more fragile, possibly by harming collagen there as well. Regulators have warned doctors to avoid these drugs in people already at risk for aneurysms unless there is no better option. The danger is rare, but the consequence is severe. Abdul's family was stunned to learn that a common antibiotic might have played a part in his crisis. He lived to tell his grandchildren to ask questions about every pill.

When the Germs Learn Back

Not every surprise looks like a tear or a rupture. While Sarah, Bruce, and Abdul each faced uncommon—even freakish—side effects of antibiotics, another man named Jacob Dye experienced a more predictable consequence of our worldwide dependence on these drugs—one that is becoming alarmingly common. Jacob was a thirty-three-year-old teacher and amateur musician. He lived a low-key life in a medium-sized city and loved taking his dog, Max, on weekend hikes.

One Saturday morning, Max tugged on the leash abruptly, causing Jacob to trip and scrape his elbow on the bark of a fallen log. It was a minor scratch, nothing a Band-Aid and some disinfectant couldn't handle. Jacob washed the cut, covered it, and thought little more of it. But unseen to him, a tiny colony of bacteria had taken root in the wound.

Over the next couple of days, Jacob started feeling under the weather: a slight fever, fatigue, and a throbbing pain radiating from that seemingly trivial scrape. By Monday, his arm was red and swollen, and he felt delirious. His wife drove him to the hospital, where doctors immediately started intravenous antibiotics. They suspected sepsis, a body-wide infection, and they were racing against time to find a drug that worked. But hour after hour, Jacob wasn't responding. The infection was raging, his blood pressure dropping. In the ICU, he heard hushed phrases like "superbug" and "resistant infection" through the fog of his fever. At one point, struggling to stay conscious, Jacob saw his distraught family through the glass and wondered if he would ever walk out of that hospital.

After a battery of tests, the hospital lab identified the culprit in Jacob's bloodstream: a strain of bacteria resistant to virtually every antibiotic the doctors had thrown at it. This "superbug," as the media often call it, was impervious to the usual cures. Each antibiotic that was meant to be a silver bullet had little effect, as if the bacteria were shrugging off the medications. The physicians turned to an old antibiotic as a last resort—a potent drug with harsh side effects, one that in a different era might have been considered too toxic except in dire emergencies. They administered it, and, in the nick of time, it worked. Jacob's fever broke. The bacteria finally began to clear from his body, not because the drug was exceptionally gentle, but because it was the microbial equivalent of a sledge-hammer. Jacob woke up days later, weak but alive, with his elated family at his side. His recovery was slow; the infection and the drugs to fight it had both taken a toll.

When he was well enough to understand, the doctors explained how precarious his case had been. The bacterium from the dog scratch had likely been a strain that evolved to resist common antibiotics, perhaps a strain of *Pseudomonas* picked up from the environment that had learned to survive our best medicines. Jacob realized with a shudder that if that last-resort antibiotic hadn't been available, he might not have survived at all. The thought that a simple scratch could lead to a near-fatal illness in the twenty-first century was sobering. It sounded like a throwback to the pre-antibiotic era, when even minor wounds could become death sentences. Yet it was not the 1920s; it was happening in 2025 "I'm living proof that the antibiotic era is beginning to crack," Jacob said later. "The drugs I always took for granted almost didn't save me. One day, they might not save the next person at all. "

107 Slow Poison: The Cost of Long-Term Use

Jacob's brush with a superbug is part of a much larger story that is unfolding worldwide. Over the past decades, bacteria have been evolving defenses against the very antibiotics designed to kill them. Each time we use an antibiotic, whether to treat a serious infection or even when antibiotics are misused for viral illnesses where they do nothing, we apply pressure on bacteria to adapt. The hardy survivors pass on their resistant traits, building armies of antibiotic-resistant bacteria. This isn't a distant theoretical threat; it's already here. A landmark study published in 2022 revealed that, in 2019, at least 1.27 million people around the world died because of infections that no antibiotic could effectively treat. In other words, antibiotic-resistant infections are killing more people each year than many major cancers. Health officials now rank antibiotic resistance as one of the top public health threats facing humanity. The problem is so pressing that the World Health Organization has called it a "silent pandemic. "

Superbugs like the one that struck Jacob are evolving faster than we can develop new drugs. Common infections, such as pneumonia, wound infections, and urinary tract infections, are gradually becoming harder to cure. In the United States alone, bacteria resistant to multiple drugs cause over 2.8 million infections each year, leading to more than 35,000 deaths annually. Globally, if current trends continue, experts warn the death toll could soar dramatically. A United Nations–backed report projected that, by 2050, as many as 10 million people per year could die from drug-resistant infections if left unchecked, a figure that commentators noted would surpass the current annual global deaths from cancer.

The stories in this chapter stretch across borders. Sarah's breathing tightened in Amsterdam. Bruce's tendon snapped in California. Abdul's artery tore in Karachi. Jacob faced a superbug in Melbourne. Different people. Different bodies. The thread is the same. Each trusted a familiar pill to help, then met an unexpected cost.

We have long treated antibiotics like a cure-all. We reach for them at the first sign of infection, and we give them to animals to prevent disease. In doing so, we have missed the quieter harms. A lung scar that never quite heals. A tendon that fails. A blood vessel wall that weakens. A microbe that learns to shrug off the very drugs we depend on.

The title of the chapter, "Slow Poison," is not about demonizing these vital drugs, but rather highlighting the slow, cumulative dangers that have lurked in their shadow. Each story in this chapter carries a lesson written in pain and perseverance. They urge a reckoning with how we use antibiotics and how we heed their risks. If there is one thread of hope running through them, it is that awareness can spur change. Sarah, Bruce, Abdul, and Jacob all turned their ordeals into cautionary tales for others, not to instill fear, but to cultivate respect for the medications that have reshaped medicine. In the end, the paradox of antibiotics is that the very tools we created to protect life must be used with care and humility, lest they become the architects of new tragedies. The slow poison of unintended consequences can be mitigated, but only if we listen to these stories and resolve to do better, before the cure becomes more dangerous than the disease.

When the Cure Steals the Sound

Christine Daglio kept a tiny notebook by the kitchen window where she wrote down the first bird she heard each morning. Robin in April. Wren in May. It was her ritual before coffee, a small joy that marked the seasons. Then, one Tuesday, she noticed the page stayed blank.

The street seemed hushed. The kettle clicked, but she did not hear it sing. Later, the radio moved her only by memory. Her favorite song lit up the dial, yet there was no chorus, only a faint, distant hum.

At her follow-up visit, she sat in a booth wearing over-sized headphones, pressing a button when a tone was audible. Mostly, she pressed nothing. The audiologist was kind and careful with words, but the result was clear. Christine had permanent hearing loss. The infection that nearly took her life was gone. The price was the sound of it.

Gentamicin had been the turning point in her care. Her blood infection did not yield to gentler drugs, so the team used an aminoglycoside, a class known for powerful bacteria killing and a known risk to the inner ear. She remembered the consent talk about "ototoxicity," and she nodded along and signed. In the storm of fevers and IV lines, survival takes the front seat. The danger to her hearing sat quietly in the back.

Here is what happened in simple terms. Deep in the inner ear live delicate hair cells that translate vibration into signals the brain understands as sound. Gentamicin can harm these cells. The risk rises with higher doses, longer courses, and repeated treatments. Age and kidney function matter because the drug is cleared through the kidneys. Slower clearance means the inner ear sees more of the medicine for longer. Christine was fifty-nine, with diabetes and borderline kidney function. Even with proper dosing and drug level checks, a small number of people like her suffer irreversible hearing loss. Most never do. Some do. It is a hard roll of the dice.

Numbers on paper can feel distant. Some studies show very low rates of hearing damage. Others, using more sensitive tests, find that many patients lose a little hearing they barely notice at first. Real life sits between those lines, and subtle losses go unreported. For Christine, the change was not subtle.

In the weeks after her hospital stay, she moved through the world as if underwater. Her husband, Luis, learned to face her when he spoke. Their granddaughter, Alma, pressed her cheek close to be heard. Church on Sundays became a blur of moving lips and missed jokes. Christine started baking again because the recipes had no volume, and she could measure sugar with a scoop and comfort with cinnamon. She felt grateful to be alive, then guilty for resenting the silence, then angry that no one had prepared her for how lonely it would feel.

Adaptation came in small, practical steps. Hearing aids were tuned and retuned. Closed captions were always on. A sticky note by the front door read "Look first" after she missed a delivery because she never heard the knock. She joined a local support group and found relief in nods from people who understood the awkward dance of lip reading and the art of pretending you caught the punchline.

Christine still keeps the notebook by the window. Some mornings she writes "birdsong, faint." Other days, the line stays empty, and she draws a small heart instead. Life has a new soundtrack, softer and uneven, but present. Her story does not argue against using powerful antibiotics. It argues for using them with care. Short courses, when possible. Careful dosing when the kidneys are tired. Honest conversations before the first dose and check-ins while the drip runs.

Christine is far from alone. Aminoglycosides like gentamicin have been workhorses since the 1940s. They are inexpensive, fast-acting, and very effective, a trio that keeps them on carts in emergency rooms and on the World Health Organization's essential medicines list. In the United States, they are common in hospitals, from newborns with suspected sepsis to adults with severe infections. One health system counted more than 5,000 patients receiving gentamicin over four years, and more than half were children under two. Across lower resource settings, the numbers are higher still. With such wide use, even a small risk touches many lives.

Most patients finish treatment with little more than brief ringing or a temporary shift on a hearing test. A meaningful minority do not. When doctors use very sensitive testing, they find that a fifth to a third of patients show some degree of hearing loss after gentamicin treatment. In the longest, heaviest courses, the toll climbs higher. People treated for drug-resistant tuberculosis with months of injectable aminoglycosides have left therapy with hearing damage in startling numbers, nearly half in some reports. The pattern is clear. The longer and more often we use these drugs, the more harm they can cause.

Medicine has tried to blunt that edge. Hospitals limit gentamicin to the shortest course that will work, often five to seven days. Pharmacists dose by weight and kidney function. Blood levels are checked to keep the drug in a narrow target range. Audiology teams step in if treatment stretches beyond a week. These safeguards help. They do not erase the risk.

Gentamicin's injury happens inside the inner ear, and blood levels do not always predict who will be sensitive. Age and tired kidneys increase the odds. In emergencies or in clinics with few resources, careful monitoring is not always possible.

That leaves a real dilemma. A drug that can save a life today may steal a sound from tomorrow. Clinicians feel that tension every time they sign the order. Christine's case makes it concrete. Her infection was cured, but her hearing was not. As her doctor said, they healed the illness and hurt the person in the same breath. That truth is the work ahead: to use powerful antibiotics with precision, to shorten courses when we can, and to treat every prescription as both a help and a hazard until we are sure which way the balance will tip.

Ken Rogers—The Price of Vision

Ken Rogers liked mornings slow and tidy. He brewed dark coffee in a dented percolator, circled the crossword in pencil, and watered the fern his students had given him when he retired from teaching history. The routine steadied him, even as a stubborn infection in his spine kept tugging at the edges of his life. He had already endured surgeries and a parade of IV antibiotics. The germ survived them all.

Linezolid felt like a small miracle. No more tubes or pumps, just pills at home. Within weeks, his back loosened and his lab numbers drifted in the right direction. He told his wife, Marla, that it felt like the first bell of the school day, the moment when chaos gives way to order. They dared to imagine a summer without hospitals.

Around week seven, the world shifted by a shade. The crossword's black squares looked washed to gray. Headlines blurred at the edges. The blue mug he loved seemed a little less blue. He joked that he needed new glasses, then squinted at the sky one afternoon and winced as if someone had turned the sun up a notch. In the living room, he clicked on an extra lamp and asked, half-teasing, half uneasy, "Did we buy a dimmer bulb, or is it me? "

At his next visit, Ken's infectious diseases doctor stopped shuffling papers. Linezolid, she explained gently, can injure the optic nerve, especially when it is taken for longer than a month. The risk is uncommon, but it is real, and it hides in long courses the way a slow leak hides under floorboards. The early clues match what Ken felt: colors fading, sharpness lost, light suddenly harsh.

The decision landed like a stone. Keep the drug and risk his sight, or stop it and risk the infection roaring back. Ken thought of his classroom windows, the way morning light used to pour across rows of desks. He thought of Marla's face in that same light. "I'll take my chances with the germ," he said, surprising himself that he could say that.

They stopped linezolid that day and rushed him to an eye specialist. The tests showed changes consistent with toxic optic neuropathy, but early, which mattered. With this kind of injury, time is everything. Remove the insult, and nerves can recover. Wait, and the damage can seal into permanence.

The next weeks were an exercise in patience and faith. Ken counted small victories. The crossword letters darkened. The blue mug returned to blue. He could read the church bulletin without holding it to his nose. In parallel, his doctors watched his spine like hawks, switched him to a different regimen, and checked his blood for quiet signs of the infection's return. It never came. By three months, his vision had largely returned with new glasses, and the ache in his back was essentially gone.

Later, Ken learned how close he had come to a different ending. Linezolid's warnings focus on food and drug interactions, but the risk to vision grows with time, dose, and a body already under strain. Not everyone rebounds, even when the drug is stopped quickly. Some lose more, and some lose everything. He felt lucky, and shaken, and a little angry at the thinness of the handouts he'd been given.

He adjusted his mornings. He still brewed coffee and watered the fern, but now he placed his glasses on the crossword and sat for a breath before he began. He kept a list in his pocket for doctor visits, the questions he wished he had asked the first time. How long will I be on this? What will we watch to make sure it is not hurting me? What is the plan if I start to notice changes?

Ken never became an activist, but he became a careful storyteller. At potlucks and barbershops, he would say, "Linezolid helped me, and it almost cost me my sight. Both can be true." He was not warning people away from strong antibiotics. He was inviting them to use strong medicine the way a good teacher uses a hard lesson—with attention, limits, and a plan to check who might be falling behind.

The fern on the windowsill grew a little lopsided that summer, reaching toward the light. Ken smiled when he noticed. He was doing the same.

Linezolid is modern medicine's sharpest kind of tool, helpful and hazardous at once. When it arrived in the early 2000s, it opened a new front against hard-to-kill germs like MRSA and VRE (vancomycin-resistant enterococci). The bonus was freedom from IV poles. Its pills work as well as an infusion, which is why Ken could go home instead of living in a hospital room.

That same strength is where the trouble hides. Short courses, a week or two, rarely cause problems, but when given for months, it does. Linezolid kills bacteria by blocking them from making proteins. In our cells, though, tiny energy makers called mitochondria use similar machinery. Over time, the drug can sap the optic nerve's power supply. The optic nerve is often the first to complain. Blurry print. Colors that fade. Light that stings. Bone marrow can falter, too. About a third of people on long courses see their blood counts slip, most often platelets, which means easy bruising and more fatigue. Ken's weekly labs told the story before his eyes did. His platelets dipped, his red cells slid, and he felt wrung out.

These side effects are tied more to time than to dose. Even the standard 600 mg twice daily can turn risky if it continues. Vision trouble tends to rise after a month and spikes around four to five months. Platelets usually begin dropping after two weeks. Older age, tired kidneys, and longer treatment raise the odds. Ken had the trifecta, which is why his team built a safety net around him: frequent blood counts, checks on his vision, and a plan to shorten or stop the moment danger appeared. Some experts will reduce the dose to once daily when the infection quiets down, hoping to spare nerves and marrow. In Ken's case, the early blur was the stop sign. His doctors halted the drug, switched to an older IV antibiotic as backup, and gave supportive vitamins while his body healed. Three months later, his vision was back to baseline with new glasses, and the infection stayed down.

The emotional toll ran alongside the lab numbers. Ken had already traded hikes for heating pads. When the edges of the world grew dim, fear did the rest. When his sight returned, relief gave way to purpose. He asked sharper questions and pressed for more explicit warnings.

Ken's case is not rare in the places where linezolid now does its hardest work. Around the world, it has become a backbone drug against multidrug-resistant tuberculosis, often taken for six months or more. In those long battles, nerve injuries add up. Reports from clinics in Europe, Africa, and South America describe many patients developing tingling in the feet, vision changes, or both. Some have to stop early because the choice becomes stark: finish the cure or keep their sight.

Medicine is adjusting. Doctors limit duration when they can, check eyes and blood on a schedule, and warn patients from day one to speak up about dimmer colors, fuzzy print, or pins-and-needles in hands and feet. New relatives of linezolid, like tedizolid, may prove gentler for long courses, but we are still learning.

Ken likes to say the drug that saved him almost blinded him, and it's true. The lesson is not to step away from powerful antibiotics. It is to step toward them with a plan. Start with the narrowest regimen that works. Set a finish line. Measure along the way. And most of all, listen to the person taking the pills because the first warning often arrives as a sentence no test can print: "The page looks dim today. "

Miguel Santos—The Sound of Sacrifice

By six a.m., Manila was already singing. Jeepneys rattled past sari-sari stores, vendors called out taho, and roosters kept time from a side alley. Miguel sat on the concrete steps and watched the city warm up. He could see the music in every gesture, but he could not hear a note. He was thirty-four, cured of tuberculosis, and living in silence.

A year earlier, Miguel had been diagnosed with multi-drug-resistant TB. Back then, the standard regimen in the Philippines still leaned on a daily injectable aminoglycoside, usually amikacin, alongside handfuls of pills. He drove a taxi by day and reported to the TB clinic before dawn, rolling up a sleeve for the shot that burned its way into the muscle. *"Laban lang,"* he told himself. Keep fighting.

Three months in, a high, unrelenting ringing followed him to bed. Tests showed his hearing was already slipping at the highest tones. The team faced a cruel math. Continue amika-cin: protect his life. Stop amikacin: protect his ears. He chose a narrow path in between, continuing a little longer while the doctors adjusted what they could. The ringing swelled, then the world went soft. One morning, he looked up, expecting the clinic's chatter, and realized the room was a movie with the sound off. Amikacin was stopped that day, and pills carried him the rest of the way.

When the doctor finally mouthed, *Mabuti,* "good news," Miguel read it on her face. He went home cured, relieved, and grieving. His son tugged his sleeve instead of shouting "Papa." His wife learned to write quick notes and tap his shoulder before speaking. Manila's streets were suddenly dangerous without the warning of horns, so he gave up the taxi. He found Filipino Sign Language classes and, to his surprise, a small circle of TB survivors who understood the price he had paid.

Miguel's story belongs to a specific moment in global health. For years, injectables like amikacin were the backbone of MDR-TB therapy, and too many patients finished treatment with permanent hearing loss. That era is fading. Since 2018, the World Health Organization has pushed programs toward all-oral regimens built around newer drugs like bedaquiline, with injectables reserved only for special cases and with strict hearing checks. Countries that switched early have already seen fewer patients leaving clinics into a silent world.

Change arrived late for Miguel, but not too late for others. His advocacy with a local NGO helped speed the adoption of all-oral treatment in his district. Miguel does not regret choosing life. On quiet mornings, he watches his children play tumbang preso in the alley and feels the city's rhythm in their laughter, even if he cannot hear it.

His story is not an argument against strong medicine. It is a plea to use it in ways that spare what makes survival sweet. In the Philippines and far beyond, that means finishing the shift to all-oral TB cures and making sure consent is more than a signature. It is a conversation, in any language, about the cost of getting well.

But sometimes the cost is not the antibiotic itself. Sometimes it is the way we deliver it.

Outpatient parenteral antibiotic therapy, or OPAT, has become the modern compromise: hospital-strength antibiotics without the hospital. For many patients, it is a bridge back to normal life. For some, it becomes a new doorway for harm. Tanya Brooks can tell you all about it.

OPAT: When the Hospital Comes Home
Tanya Brooks: The Line That Followed Her

Tanya Brooks was ready to be done with fluorescent lights.

She had been in the hospital for nine days, long enough to learn the soundtrack by heart: the soft beep of the IV pump, the shuffle of night nurses' shoes, the distant cough that seemed to echo down every hallway at three in the morning. Her infection was finally bending. The fevers had stopped. The redness on her leg had faded from angry crimson to a tired pink. The bacteria had cleared from her blood. She could sleep without waking to chills.

On discharge morning, a nurse walked in carrying a clear plastic bag that looked like a small grocery haul. Saline flushes. Alcohol caps. Tape. A thick booklet with tiny print. A box of antibiotic supplies that Tanya would store in her kitchen like an odd new pantry item.

Then the nurse lifted Tanya's sleeve.

The PICC (peripherally inserted central catheter) line sat in her upper arm, a pale tube disappearing under a clear dressing. The nurse touched the edge of the bandage and said gently, like this was normal, "This is how you'll finish your treatment."

Tanya nodded. She had heard the words already, but hearing them in the daylight made them land differently.

Outpatient parenteral antibiotic therapy. OPAT. It sounded clean and efficient. It sounded like freedom.

The infectious diseases doctor came by a few minutes later and framed it as good news. "This way you don't have to stay here for weeks," she said. "You can heal at home. We'll see you in clinic. We'll check labs. You'll have a visiting nurse. Most people do very well. "Most people.

Tanya signed the paperwork. She practiced the flush once while a nurse watched. Clamp. Scrub. Push. She was careful, the way people are careful when they know they are holding something important and breakable.

When her sister pulled up to the entrance, Tanya walked out slowly with her overnight bag and the box of supplies on her lap like a fragile package. The July air felt thick and alive. The parking lot smelled like hot asphalt and relief.

At home, the first day passed in a blur of small victories. Tanya sat on her own couch. She ate her own food. She slept without interruptions. In the morning she could hear her neighbor's lawn mower and the distant laughter of kids on bikes. Normal life, returning in pieces.

The home infusion nurse arrived at noon and turned Tanya's living room into a mini clinic. She cleaned a spot on the table. She opened sterile packaging with the calm confidence of someone who has done this a thousand times. She repeated the rules: *Keep it dry, keep it clean, watch for redness, pain, drainage, fever.* She said, "If anything feels off, you call. "

Tanya listened hard, but her mind kept wandering to the same thought: *I'm home. I made it.*

That night she showered with her arm wrapped in plastic like a cast. She moved carefully, protecting the dressing from water, and felt the strange tension of being both patient and caretaker at the same time. When she climbed into bed, the line tugged slightly, a quiet reminder that the hospital had not fully released her.

By day four, the routine had settled in. Antibiotic in the morning. Flush. Clamp. Clean and Tape. Tanya began to time her life around it the way she used to time it around school drop-offs and work shifts. Treatment became another obligation, another box to check.

That afternoon, she noticed her arm looked different.

It wasn't dramatic. Not a swollen balloon. Not a glaring emergency. Just a subtle fullness above the elbow, the kind of change you might explain away if you wanted to be done thinking about medical problems. Tanya told herself she had slept on it wrong. She lifted a grocery bag and felt a dull ache that didn't match the weight.

She pressed a finger into the skin and watched the indentation linger a beat longer than it should.

Later, during the infusion, she felt a faint warmth creep up her chest. Then a shiver. Then another. She pulled a blanket up over her shoulders and sat still, trying to decide whether this was fear or fever. Her teeth clicked once, then again. The room suddenly felt too quiet, as if her body had turned the volume down on the world.

She found the thermometer in the bathroom drawer, the one she hadn't used since her kids were small. 100.8°F. Then 101.3°F.

Tanya stared at the numbers like they were accusing her.

The nurse's words replayed in her head. *If anything feels off, you call.*

She didn't want to call. Calling meant the spell might break. Calling meant the hospital could pull her back into its orbit. Calling meant admitting that the cure still had teeth. But the chills kept coming, stronger now, rolling through her ribs. Her arm throbbed in a slow, insistent way. The dressing over the PICC looked unchanged, clean and sealed, which almost made it worse. If nothing looked wrong, why did she feel wrong?

She called anyway.

By the time she reached the emergency department, Tanya had the familiar wristband again. Blood cultures. A chest X-ray. Ultrasound of the arm. Several questions asked: "When did this start?" "Any drainage?" "Any trouble flushing the line?" The triage nurse looked at the PICC and then at Tanya's face, reading her fear.

The ultrasound tech paused longer than usual over the vein.

A doctor came in and said the word Tanya hadn't expected: "clot."

A blood clot in the arm vein that held the PICC line. A traffic jam in the vessel, built around the foreign plastic. It explained the swelling. It explained the ache. And it raised a new question: Was the fever from the infection coming back, or from bacteria hitching a ride on the line itself?

They admitted her again.

Tanya lay in a bed that wasn't hers, watching an IV drip she thought she had escaped. The box of home supplies sat untouched back at her house, a mute symbol of a plan that had looked perfect on paper.

OPAT had brought her freedom. It had also brought a new doorway for harm.

Why OPAT Exists

OPAT is one of modern medicine's best ideas. It was born from a simple truth: Hospitals are not safe places to live.

The longer someone stays in a hospital, the more they risk delirium, falls, sleep deprivation, new infections, and the slow loss of strength that comes from days spent in bed. When a patient is stable, sending them home can often be the kindest treatment we offer. It returns people to their families, their routines, and their dignity.

And for many infections, IV antibiotics really do need weeks. Bone infections. Endocarditis. Deep abscesses. Hardware infections that can't be fully removed. There are times when short and simple is not an option.

So OPAT became a bridge: hospital-level antibiotics delivered in real life.

But every bridge has weight limits. OPAT works best when we name the risks clearly, build a safety net on purpose, and decide early what would let us step down to pills instead.

That is where the hidden harms begin.

The Hidden Risks: Line, Labs, and Life at Home

On paper, OPAT looks like the perfect compromise. You treat a serious infection with serious medicine, but you do it without trapping someone in a hospital bed.

In real life, OPAT asks an ordinary person to live with an extraordinary level of medical fragility.

Because the antibiotic is only half the story. The other half is the line.

A PICC line is not just a tube. It is a foreign object sitting in a vein, crossing the border between the outside world and the bloodstream. It is a doorway. Most days, nothing happens. On the days it does, the consequences move fast.

The line

The first harm is mechanical and quietly common: the line stops behaving.

A catheter can kink. It can clot. It can slip a few centimeters without anyone noticing. A dressing that looks "fine" can loosen at the edges just enough to invite bacteria underneath. A line that flushes easily one day can meet resistance the next, and that resistance can be the first sign of a clot building around plastic.

For patients, it often starts with a small inconvenience that does not feel like medicine at all.

The infusion takes longer than usual. The arm feels "tight. "

The shoulder aches the way it does after sleeping wrong.

The infusion nurse can fix it, they hope. A little repositioning. A different angle. A flush. Another attempt.Sometimes that is all it is. Sometimes it is not.

When a clot forms in the vein, it does not announce itself with a siren. It announces itself the way many medical complications do: with vague discomfort that a tired person can rationalize away. But the danger is not vague. A clot can extend. It can inflame the vein. It can seed bacteria. In some cases, it can embolize and travel.

And then there is the fear OPAT never advertises: a line infection.

When bacteria colonize a catheter, they do not have to fight through skin and tissue the way they would in a normal infection. They have a shortcut. They can ride straight into the bloodstream. That is why the symptoms can be so dramatic, so out of proportion to what the arm looks like. A patient can have a clean dressing and still have rigors, fever, and a blood pressure that starts to dip.Clinicians know this pattern. Patients do not.

Patients often blame themselves. They replay every step. *Did I scrub long enough? Did I touch it? Did I shower wrong? Did I miss a dose?* OPAT quietly turns responsible adults into anxious detectives in their own homes.

The labs

The second hidden risk is not the line. It is what the antibiotic does while it is working.

When antibiotics are given for days, many side effects are tolerable. When they are given for weeks, side effects become a lottery with time as the ticket.

The longer the course, the more important it becomes to monitor what the body is doing in response.

This is where OPAT often looks safest in theory and becomes most fragile in practice.

In the hospital, labs happen because the system is built for it. Blood is drawn on schedule. Results populate the chart. Abnormal values trigger alarms, protocols, and consults.

At home, labs happen only if a long chain of people and steps all line up correctly. The order has to be written.

The home nurse has to come on the right day. The specimen has to be handled correctly.

The lab has to process it.

The result has to reach someone who recognizes it as abnormal. That person has to reach the patient.

Then the plan has to change in time. That is a lot of links.

And OPAT is one of the few areas in medicine where a single weak link can quietly undo the whole safety plan.

When monitoring breaks down, the harms look familiar because they are the same harms you have already explored in this book, just wearing a different mask.

Kidney function drifts downward until the dose becomes too high. Liver enzymes rise while the patient assumes fatigue is just "recovery. "

Blood counts drop slowly enough that bruising feels like clumsiness and shortness of breath feels like deconditioning.

Electrolytes change in a way that raises arrhythmia risk, and the first warning is a dizzy spell that is blamed on not eating.

OPAT can be safe. But OPAT cannot be casual. The phrase "We'll check labs" sounds reassuring in a clinic note. In a kitchen, it is a promise that needs infrastructure to keep.

Life at home

The third set of harms is the hardest to measure because it does not live in a lab value. It lives in time.

OPAT changes the rhythm of a household. It reshapes days around dosing schedules. It teaches people to count hours between infusions the way parents count hours between diapers. It forces patients to carry the hospital mindset into spaces that were supposed to represent rest.

A few weeks of OPAT can mean:

- missed work or reduced hours
- childcare rearrangements
- lost income that is never coded as a complication
- copays for supplies that arrive in intimidating boxes
- time spent on the phone coordinating deliveries, visits, and lab appointments
- the quiet embarrassment of asking a spouse or adult child to help with something that feels invasive

It can also mean isolation. A patient who is home is often treated as if they are well. Friends stop checking in. Employers expect a quick return. Family assumes normal life is back.

But OPAT is not normal life. It is medical life relocated.

Even the simplest parts have a kind of weight. Showering becomes a strategy. Clothing choices change. Sleep positions change. A simple itch under the dressing becomes a debate: ignore it or risk touching it. A child's hug becomes a moment of protective calculation.

And then there is the emotional whiplash that Tanya experienced: the feeling of freedom, followed by the sudden realization that freedom has conditions.

When OPAT goes wrong, patients often feel they have failed. They did the steps. They kept things clean. They followed instructions. And still they end up back in a hospital bed wearing another wristband.

The truth is more sobering and more honest.

Most OPAT complications are not moral failures. They are system failures, biology, and probability.

The best way to respect OPAT is to stop pretending it is simple.

The two kinds of OPAT harm

When you zoom out, OPAT harms fall into two categories.

The first category is direct: The line itself causes a new problem.

Clot. Infection. Mechanical failure. Bleeding. Accidental dislodgement. A trip to the emergency department because the line will not flush and no one knows whether it is safe to push.

The second category is indirect: The antibiotic causes a problem because monitoring is imperfect.

Kidney injury that would have been caught earlier in the hospital. Liver injury that is mistaken for fatigue.

A drug level that drifts too high. A blood count that drops quietly.An interaction that a rushed discharge summary does not fully flag.Both categories create the same ending: The patient comes back.

Not because OPAT is a bad idea, but because OPAT is a powerful idea that requires careful handling.

The question we do not ask early enough

There is one question that changes OPAT from a default plan into a deliberate one. Not "Can we send them home? "

But "Do they need to be on IV at all, and for how long? "

This is where the best OPAT programs distinguish themselves. They treat IV therapy as a phase, not a lifestyle. They plan the exit at the same time they plan the start.

Sometimes the best stewardship decision is not about withholding antibiotics. It is about choosing the safest route and the shortest effective duration.

Sometimes the safest antibiotic is not a different drug. Sometimes it is the same drug, taken by mouth.

And sometimes the most compassionate plan is not to send the hospital home at all, but to bring the treatment back to human scale.

That is why OPAT needs a safety net that is intentionally built, not merely assumed.

The Safety Net: Monitoring That Actually Works

If OPAT is going to be safe, safety cannot be a vague promise. It has to be a plan that survives real life.

Most patients hear, "We'll check labs," and picture something automatic, like an oil-change light that comes on when something is wrong. But OPAT does not come with automatic warnings. It comes with appointments, phone calls, and people. The safety net works only when everyone knows what to watch for and what happens when the numbers change. A good OPAT plan has four parts.

1) A calendar, not a suggestion

"Weekly labs" is not a plan. It is a phrase.

The patient should leave the hospital with an actual schedule: which day labs will be drawn, who will draw them, and who will call with results. Not "sometime next week," but Tuesday. Not "the nurse," but a name or a service. Not "we'll follow it," but a number to call if no one does.

Because the most dangerous OPAT complication is the one that grows quietly in the gap between intentions and execution.

2) One person owns the results

OPAT fails when everyone thinks someone else is watching.

The hospital team assumes the infusion company will notice. The infusion company assumes the clinic will notice. The clinic assumes the primary doctor will notice. The patient assumes the system will notice.

A safety net needs ownership. One clinician or one team must be clearly responsible for reviewing labs and acting on them. When that ownership is explicit, small problems stay small.

When it is not, a rising creatinine becomes a kidney injury before anyone adjusts a dose. A falling white count becomes a dangerous neutropenia before anyone pauses the drug.

3) "Red flags" that do not require medical training

The patient cannot be the only guardian of the line, but the patient is the one living with it.

So the red flags have to be simple, concrete, and repeatable. Not a paragraph of fine print. A short list on a single page that can live on the refrigerator.

Call the same day if you have:
- fever or chills, especially shaking chills
- new arm swelling, pain, or a heavy, tight feeling on the PICC side
- redness, drainage, or a dressing that lifts at the edges
- a line that will not flush easily or suddenly feels different
- new rash, hives, mouth sores, or facial swelling
- severe diarrhea, especially if watery or frequent

Go now if you experience:
- trouble breathing, chest pain, fainting, confusion
- severe weakness, severe dizziness, or a rapid heartbeat that feels wrong

These are not meant to scare patients. They are meant to keep patients from talking themselves out of seeking help when help is exactly what prevents catastrophe.

4) A planned exit, written down

The most important part of OPAT safety is not what you do on day one. It is what you plan to do on day seven.

A safe OPAT course includes a clear "step-down" conversation before discharge: If the patient improves and labs stay stable, when will we switch to oral antibiotics? If we cannot switch, what is the earliest stop date? What imaging or clinical milestone ends the course?

Without an exit plan, OPAT has a way of stretching. A few weeks becomes "just a little longer," then longer again. The line remains. The risk remains. The monitoring becomes routine, and routine is where complacency quietly grows.

The goal is not to make OPAT complicated. It already is.

The goal is to make safety explicit enough that it can survive a busy clinic, a missed phone call, a delayed nurse visit, and a tired patient who just wants to feel normal again.

Because OPAT is not only about delivering antibiotics.

It is about delivering antibiotics without delivering a new emergency.

When Pills Are Just as Good

There is a moment in many OPAT stories when the infection is improving, the patient is stable, and the IV line is no longer doing heroic work. It is just doing work.

That is the moment to ask the question that saves people from avoidable harm:

Do we still need IV?

For years, IV therapy carried a kind of automatic authority. It felt stronger. More serious. More reliable. And sometimes it is. There are infections where IV therapy is the right choice, at least early on.

But in many common situations, the benefit of staying on IV fades quickly once a patient turns the corner. The bloodstream clears. The fever stops. Pain improves. Drainage decreases. Appetite returns. The body begins to reclaim itself.

At that point, the line starts to become the bigger threat.

Because the greatest risk of OPAT is not that the antibiotic "fails." It is that the line introduces a new complication, or the monitoring misses a developing toxicity. The medicine may be correct, but the delivery system adds danger.

Oral therapy, when appropriate, removes the doorway.

No dressing. No flushing. No clot risk anchored around plastic. No midnight anxiety over whether the line feels different. And as a colleague of mine loves to remind me: You save the world by reducing plastic waste. Pills are not always simpler, but they are often safer. The decision is not emotional.

It is clinical. It depends on the infection, the organism, the source control, and the patient's ability to absorb and reliably take medication. But the mindset matters.

IV should not be a default that continues until the calendar says stop. IV should be a phase with a planned handoff. A well-run OPAT plan asks early, then asks again:

- Is the patient improving in the way we expected?
- Is there an oral option that reaches the same target effectively?
- Are we continuing IV because it is necessary, or because it is familiar?

Sometimes the most powerful stewardship move is not a different drug. It is the same intention delivered in a safer form.

A Clean Finish Line

OPAT is easy to start and surprisingly hard to end.

Not because people want to stay on it, but because endings require decisions. They require someone to say, clearly, "We're done," and to mean it.

A clean finish line has three parts.

First, a clear stop date. Not "two more weeks," but a date on the calendar. Patients live better when they can see the end.

Second, a last check that matches the risk. If you are stopping because the patient is better, confirm that "better" is real. Symptoms improved. Exam improved. The one or two labs you were following are stable. If there was a marker of infection that mattered, it is moving the right way. If imaging was the endpoint, it is planned or already done.

Third, the line comes out as soon as it is no longer needed. Not "we'll keep it a few extra days just in case." "Just in case" is how lines linger. Lingering is how complications happen.

For patients, removing the line is more than a technical step. It is a psychological release.

It is the moment the hospital finally lets go.

A clean finish line is not an afterthought. It is part of respecting antibiotics and respecting the people who have to live with our plans.

And when it is done well, OPAT becomes what it was meant to be.

A bridge back to ordinary life, not a new way to get hurt on the way home.

Between Healing and Harm

Christine's quiet mornings, Ken's dimmed pages, and Miguel's silent Manila all trace the same thin line. Powerful antibiotics saved their lives, yet each paid a price. Different drugs, different continents, yet one question remains. How much are we willing to risk to be cured?

Antibiotics are not simple heroes. Used briefly and well, they are astonishing. Stretched long, or chosen without a plan, they can turn on the very people they are meant to help. That does not mean we fear them. It means we respect them. Start with a clear goal. Set a finish line. Ask what will be watched along the way.

These stories offer plain lessons. Talk early about risks when treatment may run for weeks or months. Monitor on a schedule, not by hunch. Ken's weekly blood counts and vision checks caught trouble before it became permanent. Similar vigilance can protect hearing for patients on aminoglycosides. Science will add more tools. Researchers are testing earlier hearing screens and blood markers, and simple genetic tests already identify people who should never receive certain aminoglycosides. One day, a cheek swab may tell us which antibiotics will be harmful for Christine. Until that day arrives everywhere, prudence is our best shield.

There is a more profound lesson, too. Medicine is more than defeating microbes. It is protecting the person who carries the microbe.

The cost of a cure is not only measured in pills and scans. It may be paid in sound, sight, work, and the ease of ordinary days.

Compassionate care looks past the lab report. Connect patients quickly with audiology or ophthalmology. Offer counseling after a scare. Plan for the social ripples, like Miguel leaving his taxi and learning a new language of hands.

Zoom out, and another truth comes into focus. Long courses and harsh drugs often signal that resistance has already won a few rounds. Christine's gentamicin, Ken's linezolid, and Miguel's amikacin were all chosen because easier options failed. If we waste our best medicines, we invite a future where routine infections require dangerous regimens.

Stewardship is not a slogan. It is how we keep today's successes from becoming tomorrow's tragedies.

So we end this chapter where these patients began, with courage and clarity. They accepted hard treatments to stay alive. Their stories ask us to match that courage with better choices. Use the narrowest effective drug. Keep courses short. Check for harm while we treat harm. Inform before we prescribe, and listen when a patient says, "The page looks dim," or "The room sounds different. "

Next comes the wider fight. In "A War We Are Losing," we step beyond individual rooms and into a world where bacteria are learning faster than we are changing.

The choices we make for one patient shape the landscape for everyone. If we do not act, more people will face the kind of choices no one should have to make. If we do, the cure can remain a blessing, not a slow poison.

Key ideas
- Weeks to months of therapy multiply risks: toxicity, interactions, *C. diff.*
- Route matters: OPAT adds line risk and makes monitoring failures more costly.
- Long courses need goals, monitoring, and a finish line.

Do this — Readers
- Keep a simple calendar: doses, labs, symptoms (and line care if on OPAT).
- Ask: "What labs? How often? Who reviews them?" and "Who calls me?"
- If on OPAT: fever/chills, new arm swelling/pain, redness/drainage, or a line that won't flush = call same day.

- Revisit every one to two weeks: "Still needed?" and "When can we switch or stop?"

Do this — Clinicians
- Define targets and a stop rule up front, including IV-to-oral criteria.
- For OPAT, assign one owner for labs/line issues/dose changes.
- Schedule labs and follow-ups before discharge; don't rely on "we'll check."
- Step down to oral when appropriate; don't extend IV by default.

Conversation starters
- "What's our goal and stop rule?"
- "If I'm going home on IV antibiotics, who owns my labs and line issues, and what's the fastest way to reach them?"
- "Can any of this be done by mouth instead of intravenously? Now or soon?"

For the everyday side effects that push people to quit early or self-treat, see the Bonus Chapter: "Small Harms, Big Consequences." You can also visit *beyondthecurebook.com* for a checklist.

Chapter 9

A War We Are Losing

The President's Son (1924)

On a warm June afternoon in 1924, a sixteen-year-old boy named Calvin played tennis on the White House lawn. He darted across the clay court in his canvas shoes, laughing as he tried to return his older brother's serve. In the excitement, Calvin hadn't worn socks, and by the end of the match, a small blister had formed on his right big toe. It seemed trivial at the time, just a little bubble of skin from an hour of summertime fun. But within a few days that tiny blister would change the course of his family's life and send a chill through the entire nation.

By the next morning, Calvin's toe was swollen and throbbing. The White House physician frowned as red streaks crept up the boy's foot, a sign the infection was spreading. In 1924, doctors had few weapons against such infections. There were no antibiotics at all. Instead, they tried cleaning the wound and applied antiseptic ointments. Calvin was soon running a high fever and becoming delirious with pain. His condition worsened so rapidly that he was rushed to Walter Reed Hospital. There, some of the country's best doctors could do little but watch and hope. The infection, later described as "blood poisoning," had entered his bloodstream. What likely started as an ordinary *Staphylococcus aureus* (staph) bacteria in the blister was now raging unchecked throughout his body. In today's terms, Calvin was septicemic, his immune system overwhelmed by bacteria with no medicine to fight back.

His father, President Calvin Coolidge, kept vigil at the hospital, helplessly watching his youngest son slip away. The power of the presidency could summon generals and pass laws, but it could not command a cure that didn't exist. One week after that innocent tennis game, Calvin Coolidge Jr. died from the infection. The White House flag fluttered at half-mast as the news broke. The nation was stunned: the President's son felled by something as common as a blister. It was a heartbreaking reminder that in the era before antibiotics, even the most privileged and protected were vulnerable to sudden, lethal infections.

President Coolidge was shattered. He later confided that "when he [Calvin Jr.] went, the power and the glory of the Presidency went with him." Losing his son broke him in a way no political crisis ever could. At a time when America was roaring through the Jazz Age, reveling in prosperity and progress, this tragedy exposed a frightening truth: Modern civilization was still at the mercy of microscopic germs. A simple scrape or sore throat could turn into a death sentence, and doctors were essentially empty-handed in the face of aggressive bacteria. It was a war for survival, and in 1924, humanity was losing battle after battle. Little did anyone know, relief was on the horizon, but so was a new chapter of that war, one that is still unfolding today.

The First Miracle (1942)

Less than two decades later, the world was mired in another crisis—World War II—but a medical miracle was quietly brewing in the background. In March 1942, inside a Connecticut hospital room, a thirty-three-year-old woman named Anne Miller lay at death's door. Anne was a nursing school graduate and the wife of a Yale University athletic director. Normally healthy and energetic, she had suffered a miscarriage that winter and then developed a severe infection afterward. The infection spread into her bloodstream, and like Calvin Coolidge Jr., Anne was stricken with life-threatening septicemia, or "blood poisoning," as it was still commonly called. For weeks, her fever soared above 106°F (41°C). Nurses packed her in ice to try to bring the fever down, and doctors threw everything they had at the infection. They transfused her with blood. They performed surgeries to drain abscesses. They administered the best drugs available at the time, including the new sulfa drugs, which were the first antibiotics discovered in the 1930s.

Nothing worked. Anne's infection was too severe. After a month in the hospital, she was delirious, her weight dropping, her body exhausted by constant fever. The medical team had run out of options and was preparing for the worst.

Unbeknownst to most people, a revolutionary cure had been discovered in England just a few years earlier: penicillin. It was a substance derived from a humble mold, and it had the astonishing ability to kill bacteria. However, in early 1942, penicillin was still experimental and incredibly scarce. Producing even a tiny amount was difficult and time-consuming; growing enough of the "mold juice" to treat one person took enormous effort and resources. Most of the world had never heard of it. But Anne Miller's doctor had a desperate idea. Through a colleague's connection, he learned that a group of scientists in Britain and the United States was working to make penicillin available, and a tiny supply might exist for special cases. Anne certainly qualified as special—she was on the brink of death, with an infection nothing else could cure.

The doctor sent out an urgent plea. In the midst of wartime, U.S. authorities controlled vital medical supplies, and penicillin was as precious as gold. Miraculously, the request was approved. A small quantity of penicillin, about a table-spoon's worth, roughly half of the entire available stock of penicillin in the United States at that time, was rushed to New Haven Hospital for Anne. On March 14, 1942, nurses injected the pale yellow fluid into Anne Miller's veins and then held their breath. What happened next would become the stuff of medical legend. Within twenty-four hours, Anne's raging fever broke. The color returned to her cheeks. In a few days, this woman who had been hovering at death's door opened her eyes, smiled, and started to recover. The penicillin was like a magic bullet, obliterating the bacteria that had made her so ill. Anne Miller's life had been saved by a new kind of miracle drug.

Unfortunately, a year earlier, another patient wasn't as lucky. Albert Alexander, a forty-three-year-old British police officer, was the first human to be treated with penicillin. What began as a simple scratch on his face, likely from a rose thorn in his garden, spiraled into a devastating infection that claimed one of his eyes and spread rapidly through his body. In February 1941, as he hovered near death, doctors at Oxford gave him an intravenous dose of penicillin, the first ever used in a human. The results were astonishing: within a day, his fever dropped, and his condition improved dramatically. But the supply was heartbreakingly limited. The team tried to recycle the drug from his urine to extend the treatment, but after just five days, they ran out. The infection returned with a vengeance, and Alexander died a few weeks later. His brief reprieve, however, demonstrated penicillin's lifesaving power and helped ignite the antibiotic revolution.

Word of Anne's astonishing turnaround spread quickly among doctors and scientists. If penicillin could rescue a patient as sick as Anne, what else could it do? The answer, it turned out, was to revolutionize medicine. In the months and years following Anne Miller's cure, penicillin production was scaled up feverishly, driven by the urgent needs of World War II. By 1944, enough penicillin was being produced to treat wounded soldiers on the battlefields of Europe and the Pacific, and soon after, to supply civilian hospitals as well. Infections that had once been death sentences—pneumonia, infected wounds, childbirth fever—could now be treated effectively. The change was so dramatic that it's hard to overstate: The introduction of antibiotics transformed human life. Average life expectancy leaped upward as deaths from common infections plummeted. Surgeons could perform riskier operations knowing they had a tool to treat infections. Minor cuts or throat infections no longer carried the same mortal fear.

Anne Miller walked out of the hospital and went on to live a full life, eventually reaching ninety years of age. She became a living testament to the power of antibiotics. It felt as though humanity had finally gained the upper hand in the age-old war against bacteria. The wonder drugs weren't limited to penicillin, either—scientists discovered streptomycin, tetracycline, and a host of other antibiotics in the following decades. By the mid-twentieth century, a doctor encountering a dangerous infection had an arsenal of different pills and injections to choose from. For the first time in history, it seemed we might permanently defeat the microbial enemies that had haunted us for millennia. The horrors of patients dying from a cut finger or an ill-timed blister seemed destined to fade into history books, a grim reminder of a bygone era before the cure was found.

The Rising Tide of Resistance

For a time, it felt as if the story had a happy ending. A sore throat met penicillin and cleared in days. Surgeons gave a preventative dose and slept more easily. Farmers treated sick animals and added antibiotics to their food to prevent infection. Travelers packed a just-in-case prescription, and parents kept a half-finished bottle in the cabinet. Antibiotics became the quiet promise behind everyday life. If you got an infection, you took the pills and moved on.

Beneath that calm surface, the bacteria were busy. In laboratories and wards, a pattern appeared, then refused to go away. The usual drugs did not always work. Penicillin, once a lightning bolt, dulled against some staph infections. Doctors answered with methicillin.

The microbes answered in kind. Methicillin-resistant *Staphylococcus aureus* earned a new name, MRSA, and a reputation for climbing past our defenses. At first, it lingered in intensive care units and postoperative wings. Then it stepped into locker rooms, prisons, and households, carried on skin and shared towels.

The rhythm became familiar. We built a new wall. The bacteria learned where the mortar was thin. A few cells survived, passed along the trick, and turned it into a blueprint for the next generation. Resistance spread in small increments that added up. A urinary infection that once yielded to a simple drug needed something stronger. A pneumonia that used to bend in forty-eight hours held out for a week. The victories were still coming, but they were not as easy, and they did not last as long.

By the early years of the new century, superbugs were no longer a hospital rumor. Healthy people arrived at clinics with boils, skin infections, or stubborn sinusitis that shrugged at first-line antibiotics. Each case felt like a warning taped to the exam room door. The miracle had never been permanent. It had always been a race, and we had slowed our pace while the microbes kept running.

Why did they gain ground? Partly because we helped them. We used antibiotics when a virus was the real culprit. We stirred small doses into feed and water on crowded farms. Every unnecessary pill, every suboptimal dose, was a training drill for the enemy. The bacteria learned faster in the presence of our weapons, not in their absence.

The tide has not fully turned, but it is rising. The lesson is not despair. It is humility. Antibiotics remain astonishing. They also remain fragile. Treat them as a finite resource, and they will keep saving lives. Treat them as a cure-all, and they will slip from our hands, one common infection at a time.

Bob Rogers' Ordeal (Modern Day)

Bob Rogers did not picture himself as a headline for antibiotic resistance. He was fifty-two, a dad of two, and the kind of bloke who spent Saturday mornings coaching junior footy and Sunday afternoons barbecuing snapper in the backyard. He lived in a coastal suburb outside Newcastle, where the ocean rolls in heavy and blue, and the magpies argue in the Norfolk pines. A nagging knee from many years of surfing finally pushed him to book elective surgery. In Australia, this is routine. You go in, you get it fixed, you go home.

The operation went smoothly. Bob woke to the sound of kookaburras outside his ward window and a physiotherapist telling him he was already ahead of schedule. He texted a photo of the bandaged knee to his kids with the caption

"Bionic Dad." He was sent home with instructions, a packet of pain tablets, and a short course of antibiotics to keep infection at bay. For a few days, it felt like a small detour on a good road.

On day six, the detour became a bog. Bob spiked a fever. His knee turned red, hot, and tight as a drum skin. The pain cut through sleep and made him gasp. Back at the hospital, the team suspected a joint infection and started a standard antibiotic that usually sorts out the usual culprits. It did not. The fevers climbed. Night sweats soaked the sheets. His wife sat by the bed and watched the easy confidence drain from the room.

Cultures told the truth. This was staph, but not the kind that yields to first-line drugs. The lab reported resistance. The term *MRSA* entered the conversation. Bob blinked at the letters. He knew them from the news, from stories about hospital bugs in far-off places. Now the letters were on his chart. The doctors switched antibiotics, then switched again, adjusting doses while the infection pressed its advantage.

There is a sound to a ward when things turn. Monitors click more often. Voices lower. Pages come faster. Bob felt it. What began as a tidy fix had become a race. When the lab map finally pointed to a drug with a chance, the team hung a bag of vancomycin and watched every hour. It is a powerful medicine that asks the kidneys to work hard and the nurses to keep careful count. Slowly, the fevers eased. The angry heat around the knee faded from red to pink. He went to the operating theater for a washout to clear infected tissue, then back to the ward to start again.

Recovery was the long part. Weeks on an IV line. Nausea that arrived before lunch and stayed for dinner. Physiotherapy that felt like climbing sand hills. Bob made progress in small ways. First, a shuffle to the corridor. Then, a lap of the ward.

One morning, he stood at the window and watched a storm roll in from Stockton Beach, sheets of rain marching across the harbor, and he thought about how close he had come to vanishing under it.

He went home with a cane and a careful plan. The kids joked that the cane made him look like a cricket umpire. He laughed, then told them what had happened in the simplest terms he could. A common germ had learned uncommon tricks. The pills that used to work did not. He had been saved by one of the few medicines left that could still land a punch.

Amina's Story: No Borders, No Mercy

Amina's labor ended at dawn, just as the roosters began their chorus across the hills. She was twenty-seven, a market seller from a village outside Eldoret, and now a mother of two. Aunties brewed chai, neighbors arrived with maize flour, and the church women sang a soft lullaby on the veranda. For a day, it felt like every Kenyan birth story, full of bustle and blessing.

Then a slow burn started. First, a sting when she stood. Then chills that rattled her bones. By evening, a fever had settled in. At the clinic, the nurse listened, pressed a hand to Amina's belly, and suspected a postpartum infection. It is a common complication, usually handled with antibiotics. They gave what they had and told her to rest.

Two days passed with no relief. Amina could barely nurse. Her mother sent an M-Pesa (a mobile money service) request through the family group, and by afternoon, cousins had pooled enough for a hire car. The bumpy road into town shook the windows and jostled the baby to sleep. By the time they reached the referral hospital, Amina's blood pressure was dropping. That is sepsis, the body's alarm when infection spills into the blood.

In the emergency ward, the team started intravenous antibiotics and fluids. Lab results told the rest of the story. The
bacteria were resistant to the first drug. They did not flinch
for a second. The pattern was familiar to the doctors. Years of
easy access to antibiotics in chemists' shops and farm sheds
had given local microbes time to learn. What worked once
no longer did.

They tried what the pharmacy could supply. Some newer
medicines were out of stock or priced beyond a small hospital's reach. A clinician called Nairobi and secured a last-resort
antibiotic from a larger center. A boda rider took the parcel
to the bus. A night matatu carried it west.

When the vial finally reached the ward, the nurses hung
it without a word and watched the numbers on the monitor.
For a moment, the fever softened. Amina opened her eyes
and asked for her son. Then her kidneys began to fail, strained
by days of infection and strong drugs. Her skin turned cool.
In the blue light of the ward, with her husband sleeping on a
wooden bench in the corridor, Amina slipped away.

Her death was not from a rare parasite or a dramatic
injury. It was a bacterial infection that arrived at the wrong
time with the wrong resistance, in a place where the right
medicine was hard to find. Before antibiotics, stories like this
were common. The unsettling truth is that in some parts of
the world, they are becoming common again.

Antibiotic resistance does not respect borders. It grows
wherever medicines are overused or underdosed, in city hospitals and roadside clinics, in rich countries and rural counties.
Amina's village will remember her as a bright trader and a
gentle mother. Her story carries a broader lesson. Winning this
war will take more than one hospital and one family's haram-
bee. It will take careful prescribing, steady supply chains, and

the humility to treat every antibiotic as precious so that the next mother with a fever lives to hum her child back to sleep.

Van Clarde's Last Fight

Van Clarde loved the chaos of new cities. When his firm sent him from Connecticut to New Delhi for an engineering site visit, he packed a notebook, a camera, and a stubborn curiosity. He rode the metro at rush hour, ate *pani-puri* in Connaught Place, and finished late nights with masala chai from a street cart where the vendor poured it high to cool the foam. One afternoon in Old Delhi, he joined a colleague for chaat and hot jalebi, crisp and dripping, while scooters threaded past their ankles.

It felt like the world had turned upside down.

Halfway through the week, he had a brief bout of traveler's stomach, nothing dramatic, then he bounced back and flew home. He felt fine when he checked into the surgical center two weeks later for an elective hernia repair. The operation was routine. He was home that evening with instructions, pain pills, and a plan to take it easy.

On day five, his incision pulled tight and angry. A fever followed, then a deep ache that would not let go. In the clinic, the surgeon pressed gently and immediately became concerned about an abscess. They drained it and sent the fluid to the lab. Van started a broad-spectrum antibiotic that usually handles this kind of infection. It did not work. The fever climbed again.

Culture results changed the stakes. The lab had grown *Klebsiella* carrying NDM, a New Delhi metallo-beta-lactamase. In plain terms, the bacteria made an enzyme that sliced through many antibiotics, including carbapenems, which are among the strongest drugs we have. The likely story was this: In Delhi, Van had picked up the organism in his gut without knowing it. Many people carry these resistant bacteria quietly. During surgery, a few cells likely slipped into the wound, then multiplied.

The hospital moved quickly. He was placed in isolation to protect other patients. Infectious disease specialists joined the team and switched therapy to ceftazidime–avibactam, a paired drug where one component attacks the bacteria and the other shields the attack by blocking resistance mechanisms. They also focused on source control, reopening the incision to clear any remaining pockets of pus and debris. Antibiotics cannot cure what a scalpel has not reached.

The first days were tense. Van slept little, then sat up and watched snow fall past the window, flakes drifting over the parking lot, so different from the heat he remembered on Chandni Chowk. By the fourth day on the new regimen, his fever broke. The redness faded. Lab markers that had been stubborn finally bent in the right direction.

Recovery was not glamorous. Daily wound care. Almost two weeks of intravenous antibiotics delivered through a line he had to guard like a fragile wire. A food list taped to the fridge to keep his gut steady while his body healed. He returned to work later than planned, leaner and more careful with hand gel.

Van's case reads like a postcard from a connected world. A meal on a busy street, a harmless colonization in the gut, an elective surgery at home, and then a surprise: a microbe built to evade our best drugs. He did not carry a scandalous story of risk. He carried what anyone might pick up while moving through a crowded planet.

What saved him was a mix of old and new, scalpel and science, and a team that knew when to change course.

The Rise of Resistance

To understand how we arrived at this perilous point, we must rewind to the beginning of the antibiotic era. It all started in the early twentieth century with a chance discovery that changed the course of medicine. In 1928, Alexander Fleming returned from vacation to find a mold growing in one of his petri dishes. That mold, by pure luck, was killing the bacteria he had been studying. Fleming had stumbled upon penicillin, the world's first true antibiotic. When penicillin was finally mass-produced in the 1940s, it was nothing short of a miracle. Soldiers with infected wounds, once doomed to suffer or die, recovered swiftly.

Pneumonia, blood infections, and strep throat, illnesses that had been death sentences for centuries, could now be cured with a few doses of this wonder drug.

Antibiotics emerged as the magic bullet of medicine, and doctors were suddenly armed with a powerful cure for countless ailments.

In those early days, it seemed bacteria had met their ultimate defeat. But Fleming himself knew better. He famously warned that if antibiotics were used improperly, bacteria would learn to resist them. And he was right. Not long after penicillin became widely available, reports surfaced of bacteria that no longer responded to it. A stubborn strain of *Staphylococcus*, a common germ that can cause skin infections and pneumonia, had essentially shrugged off the new drug. Scientists were alarmed but not deterred. They responded by inventing new antibiotics: streptomycin, tetracycline, erythromycin, and many more joined the arsenal over the next few decades. Each time bacteria evolved to resist one drug, a new medicine was ready to take its place. For a while, it felt like we could stay one step ahead in this microbial arms race.

By the late twentieth century, however, cracks in our strategy were becoming clear. The golden age of antibiotic discovery was fading. Fewer new antibiotics were being developed, even as bacteria continued to adapt and outwit existing drugs. Doctors started encountering infections that required multiple rounds of different antibiotics to cure. In hospitals, certain bacteria developed resistance not just to one but to many drugs, earning the ominous label of "multidrug-resistant." The war had quietly begun to turn. We were using our antibiotic weapons faster than we could replace them, and the bacteria were growing stronger with each passing year.

Consider Keala Reyes, who lived on the windward side of O'ahu, Hawaii, where the Ko'olau cliffs rise like green walls and the air tastes of salt and plumeria. At forty-six, she made her living as a graphic designer, often working late into the night for local musicians. Years of smoking had narrowed her lungs, but she carried her COPD with the quiet resilience that island life can teach you. She kept promising herself she'd quit "one of these days. "

Her trouble began with a rough cough that drained her faster than usual. By the end of the week, she couldn't take ten steps without stopping to breathe. In the ICU, even high-flow oxygen barely held her up. A bronchoscopy revealed the real story: severe *Stenotrophomonas maltophilia* pneumonia, a bacterium known for evading many of the antibiotics we rely on. The lab showed it carried two enzymes—L1 and L2—that together dismantle nearly every drug aimed at them.

The first days were discouraging. Trimethoprim-sulfamethoxazole didn't help. Levofloxacin and minocycline did nothing. Keala remained ventilated and sedated while her team worked through the options.

By day six, they turned to a strategy built on resourcefulness rather than new medicines. They paired ceftazidime-avibactam (CZA) with aztreonam, two older drugs used together, as a workaround. The idea was simple: Avibactam blocks L2, which normally destroys aztreonam, and aztreonam is naturally stable against L1. When given side by side, each drug protects the other, creating an opening against an organism that usually has the upper hand.

Slowly, her numbers improved. Fevers eased. Ventilator settings dropped. One morning, as the sun rose over the Ko'olau, Keala passed her breathing trial. The tube came out. She whispered *"mahalo"* to the respiratory therapist. Thanks.

When she went home, she carried a portable oxygen tank and a new resolve. Her pulmonologist didn't lecture her about smoking; he simply reminded her that every cigarette would close the door she had just fought to reopen.

She understood. Some lessons settle in without words. Keala's recovery wasn't from a miracle drug. It came from clinicians thinking creatively and squeezing the last strength out of antibiotics that we are quickly losing. Cases like hers are appearing more often now, quiet signals that the rise of resistance is no longer theoretical. It is already shaping the way we practice medicine, one patient at a time.

The rise of antibiotic resistance was not dramatic at first; there were no explosions or sudden catastrophes to mark the shift. Instead, it crept up on us in countless small incidents: an ear infection that needed a second antibiotic to clear up, a case of tuberculosis that took months of treatment instead of weeks, a postsurgery wound that didn't heal as expected.

These were warning signs, easy to ignore individually, but together they painted a troubling picture. Humanity's wonder drugs were losing their wonder.

Quietly and persistently, bacteria were evolving into enemies we could no longer take for granted. The very medicines that once assured us easy victories were becoming less reliable year by year, patient by patient.

A Global Crisis

This is not one hospital's problem or one country's bad luck. It is a global drift toward danger. In 2019, researchers estimated that antibiotic-resistant infections killed more than 1.2 million people in a single year. That is more than HIV or malaria. Each number is a face, a family, a story that ended because the right drug no longer worked.

The burden falls hardest where resources are thin. In parts of South Asia and sub-Saharan Africa, newborns develop bloodstream infections that ignore the medicines on the shelf. Drug-resistant typhoid and tuberculosis cut down teenagers and parents in their prime. A scraped knee, a postoperative wound, a bout of diarrhea—any of these can turn dangerous if the bacteria have learned our playbook. Wealthy nations are not spared. In the United States and Europe, hospitals screen for superbugs, isolate carriers, and still see outbreaks. Routine urinary infections more often shrug at first-line pills. Some strains of gonorrhea now resist almost everything. Cancer care and organ transplantation rely on antibiotics to keep patients safe; lose those drugs, and modern medicine loses its safety net.

Health agencies are blunt about what comes next if we drift. The World Health Organization warns of a post-antibiotic era, a time when common infections and minor injuries become serious again. Some forecasts suggest that by 2050, resistant infections could claim ten million lives each year. That would make superbugs one of the world's leading killers.

This is not science fiction. It is a slow, quiet pandemic that spreads with travel, trade, and routine clinic visits. Bacteria do not care about borders, income, or intentions. The only workable answer is collective. We either protect these medicines together, with careful use and steady investment in new tools, or we watch the ground erode beneath all of us, one preventable loss at a time.

Global Snapshot

In 2015, countries agreed on a common plan to slow the spread of antimicrobial resistance; however, it remains unclear whether this plan has led to a change in behavior. A recent analysis of antibiotic sales from 2010 to 2021 offers a clear answer. Most high-income countries used fewer antibiotics as the decade went on, while many low- and middle-income countries used more. The fastest rises were seen in an eight-country group in West Africa, in China, and in Algeria. The steepest drops came from Singapore, South Africa, and Finland. These shifts matter because total use sets the stage for what resistance will look like in a few years.

The study also looked at use through the WHO's AWaRe lens. "Access" drugs are the first choices for common infections. "Watch" drugs carry a higher risk for resistance, and "Reserve" drugs are our last line when nothing else works. The WHO goal is straightforward: At least 60% of all antibiotic use should come from "Access" agents. Think of that threshold as the speed limit for safe driving. When systems meet or exceed that mark, they tend to protect future options. When they do not, they push more care into the "Watch" and "Reserve" lanes where the risks climb.

Which medicines moved the needle? Amoxicillin remained the most used antibiotic worldwide. At the same time, carbapenems (our high-end broad-spectrum antibiotics) continued to rise, with use increasing by about 54% between 2011 and 2021.

Carbapenems live in the "Watch" and "Reserve" space, so growth here is not just a statistic. It is a warning that broad-spectrum drugs are being pulled into everyday care more often than they should be.

The consequences show up in the bugs we fight every day. Places that used more antibiotics had higher resistance in *Escherichia coli, Klebsiella pneumoniae, Pseudomonas aeruginosa, Streptococcus pneumoniae, Staphylococcus aureus,* and *Enterococcus faecium*. More pressure, more resistance. For us, the path forward is practical. Start with "Access" drugs when they fit, dose them right, and set a stop date.

Track and share your "Access" percentage by service and prescriber. Place extra layers of review on carbapenems and other broad-spectrum choices.

This picture has limits, and the authors were clear about them. Sales data do not capture every prescription, and resistance rates are based on European surveillance reports rather than a single global lab network. Even with those limits, the direction and size of change are hard to ignore. The world did not move in one direction after 2015. That is why the solutions must be local, disciplined, and visible on a dashboard that anyone on the team can read.

Why Are We Losing?

By now, it is clear that antibiotic resistance isn't just a twist of fate; it is a crisis of our own making. The bacteria evolved, yes, but we humans also helped them along through our actions and inactions. How did we end up giving the advantage back to these germs?

Several key factors have tilted the balance in the bacteria's favor:

- **Overuse and misuse in human medicine:** For decades, antibiotics have been handed out too freely. Doctors often prescribed them for illnesses like colds or the flu, even though those are caused by viruses that antibiotics can't treat. Patients, too, have played a part by pressuring physicians for quick fixes or by not taking antibiotics correctly. Many people have skipped doses or stopped their antibiotic course as soon as they felt better, giving surviving bacteria a chance to regroup and become resistant. Every time an antibiotic is used unnecessarily or improperly, it's like giving bacteria a free training session to outsmart the drug.

- **Excessive use in livestock and agriculture:** Antibiotics aren't just used in people; they are also used by the ton in farming. In many countries, cows, chickens, and pigs are routinely given antibiotics to prevent illness in crowded conditions or simply to promote faster growth. This constant exposure breeds resistant bacteria on the farm. Those resistant germs can then spread beyond the farm—through the meat we eat, the soil and water polluted by animal waste, and through farm workers. A resistant bug that emerges on a poultry farm in one country can hitch a ride in undercooked meat to someone's dinner table halfway around the world.

- **Poor infection control and sanitation:** Bacteria thrive where hygiene is poor. In hospitals and clinics, if proper handwashing and sterilization practices are not strictly followed, resistant bacteria can easily hop from one patient to another. Outside of healthcare settings, lack of clean water and proper sanitation in some communities means more infections are spreading unchecked. Every infection that spreads is another infection that may need antibiotics, which in turn increases the chances of resistance. The ease of international travel today also means that a superbug in one city can quickly become a problem in another. We've created a world where bacteria can spread rapidly, but our defenses (like consistent infection-control practices) haven't kept up.

- **Fewer new antibiotics in development:** Perhaps one of the biggest reasons we are losing ground is that we aren't getting reinforcements. Developing a new antibiotic is scientifically challenging, and it's also not very profitable for pharmaceutical companies. An antibiotic is typically taken for a week or two, curing the patient, whereas drugs for chronic conditions (like heart disease or diabetes) can be taken for life, which makes them more lucrative.

Over the past few decades, most big drug companies drastically scaled back their antibiotic research programs.

- As a result, the pipeline of new antibiotics has slowed to a trickle. We are trying to fight evolving superbugs with old, aging weapons, and many of those weapons are no longer effective.

These are just a few of the factors, but these factors have combined to create a perfect storm. We have bacteria that are smarter and tougher because of our overuse of antibiotics, and we have fewer new drugs to throw at them because of our choices in medicine and policy. It's a sobering realization that we—doctors, patients, parents, farmers, policymakers—have inadvertently facilitated the threat that now looms so large.

The Stakes

What would it really mean if antibiotics stopped working? The consequences would reach far beyond just a few more sick days. In truth, the loss of antibiotics would throw us back to a time before modern medicine. Here are some of the major things at risk:

- **Routine surgeries and organ transplants:** Today, procedures like appendix removals, joint replacements, and heart surgeries are considered safe largely because antibiotics prevent or treat infections that can occur during and after the operation. If antibiotics fail, even a standard surgery could become life-threatening. Organ transplants, which require doctors to suppress the patient's immune system, would be nearly impossible because infections would run rampant with no way to control them.

- **Childbirth safety:** Not long ago, childbirth was one of the most dangerous moments in a woman's life largely because of the high risk of infection after delivery. Antibiotics changed that, drastically reducing deaths from postpartum infections and Caesarean sections. Without effective antibiotics, those risks would rise again. Mothers and newborns could once more face deadly infections in the days and weeks after birth, erasing decades of progress in maternal and infant health.

- **Cancer and other medical treatments:** Many modern medical treatments depend on antibiotics as a safety net. Cancer chemotherapy, for example, weakens the immune system, leaving patients prone to infections that are normally kept at bay. Right now, antibiotics help protect these vulnerable patients. Similarly, treatments like dialysis for kidney disease or steroid therapies for certain chronic illnesses put people at higher risk of infection. If effective antibiotics are no longer available, doctors would have to reconsider or scale back these treatments, knowing they could become too dangerous without the ability to treat infections.

- **Common injuries and infections:** Imagine a world where a scraped knee or a routine case of strep throat could kill. This was the reality for our great-grandparents. A simple cut from gardening could lead to a lethal infection like gangrene. A child's ear infection could spread and become life-threatening. We could return to that reality. Minor infections that we barely worry about today might once again turn fatal if no antibiotics can stop them. Even something as routine as a tooth extraction or a case of food poisoning could become perilous.

In short, the stakes of losing our antibiotics are almost unimaginable. We risk losing not just treatments for infections but also the trust that is essential for modern healthcare to function. Our advances in surgery, cancer therapy, intensive care, and virtually every field of medicine rely on the quiet assurance that antibiotics will be there if an infection strikes. Take that assurance away, and much of what we consider "safe" and "routine" in medicine could crumble. This is the precipice on which we now find ourselves.

Fighting Back

Hope is not a slogan here; it is a plan. Around the world, people are changing how we use the very drugs that changed history. The problem is real, the stakes are high, yet the response is gathering strength.

The first line of defense is stewardship, which simply means using antibiotics with care. Hospitals now pair prescribers with pharmacists who double-check doses and durations. Infectious diseases specialists have been empowered to gate-keep antibiotics with support from pharmacists trained in infectious diseases.

Swabs and rapid tests help confirm that an infection is bacterial before a prescription is written. When a drug is needed, the choice is narrow and precise rather than broad and indiscriminate. Family clinics are having honest conversations with patients. A cough from a virus does not need an antibiotic. This is medicine with seatbelts on.

Outside the clinic, the food chain is changing. Many countries have banned routine antibiotic use for growth promotion in livestock. Farmers are improving hygiene in barns, vaccinating herds, and using targeted treatment only when animals are sick. Supermarkets and restaurants are asking suppliers for meat raised with fewer antibiotics, and consumers are voting with their wallets. Clean water and sanitation projects add another layer of protection because the infection you never get is the antibiotic you never need.

Innovation is moving again. Scientists are mining soil, oceans, and caves for new compounds, and a few have already reached early trials. Others are reviving old ideas with modern tools, like phage therapy, which uses viruses that hunt specific bacteria. Vaccines are expanding beyond childhood schedules to prevent bacterial pneumonia, typhoid, and more.

In each case, the goal is the same: prevent infection when we can, and when we cannot, meet it with new options.

Policy is catching up to the science. More than a hundred countries have national action plans for antimicrobial resistance. Public funds and new incentive models are being built so that companies can afford to develop drugs we hope to use sparingly. Data systems now track resistance patterns across borders, letting doctors choose smarter treatments in real time. None of this is flashy; all of it matters.

These efforts are already bearing fruit. Hospitals that tightened hygiene and cut unnecessary prescriptions have seen resistant infections fall. When a vaccine against a common bacterial pneumonia rolled out, antibiotic use dropped because fewer people became ill. Small wins add up. Each avoided prescription is one less training session for a future superbug.

We should be clear-eyed. Bacteria will continue to evolve, and no one expects a final victory parade. What we can do is regain control. Use antibiotics when they help, hold back when they do not, and keep building new tools so tomorrow's doctors are not left empty-handed. Living with our microbial neighbors in balance is possible.

One idea points the way. For many infections, shorter courses work as well as longer ones, and overtreating can cause harm. Less can truly be more. Shorter treatment means fewer side effects, less disruption of the microbiome, and fewer chances for resistance to emerge, while still curing the infection in front of us. It is a simple shift with profound effects.

So the path forward is disciplined and hopeful. Stewardship at the bedside. Restraint on the farm. Clean water in every community. New drugs, new vaccines, and old tools used wisely. Most of all, a change in mindset. Antibiotics are precious, and when we treat them that way, they last.

In the next chapter, "Paradigm Shift: When Less Is More," we will explore how careful, shorter, and more innovative treatment can keep patients safe today while protecting tomorrow's cures. The war is not over. The way we choose to fight it can still change the ending.

Key ideas
- Resistance is a moving target; today's easy infection can be tomorrow's hard one.
- Personal choices aggregate into community risk.

Do this — Readers
- Vaccinate, wash hands, prepare food safely, and use condoms where appropriate.
- Take antibiotics exactly as prescribed; never request them for colds.
- Support stewardship in your hospital or clinic.

Do this — Clinicians

- Use local antibiograms; narrow/shorten by default.
- Educate at discharge about adherence and red flags.
- Report resistant organisms per policy; partner with infection prevention.
- Involve the infectious diseases doctors promptly.

Conversation starters

- "What's resistance like in our area?"
- "How do my choices affect community risk?"

Chapter 10

Paradigm Shift: When Less Is More

On a humid afternoon in Khulna, Bangladesh, the power flickered and ceiling fans slowed to a lazy spin. Sima sat on a woven charpoy, cradling her daughter, Amina, who coughed in short, tight bursts. The village pharmacy had already tried a syrup and ginger tea. None of it eased the rasp in the little girl's chest. When the neighbor's rickshaw pulled up at last, Sima wrapped Amina in a thin shawl and hurried to the upazila clinic.

The clinic was crowded, children on laps and grandparents on benches, a chorus of soft coughs and murmurs. The doctor listened to Amina's lungs and nodded, face gentle. "Pneumonia," he said. Years ago, he would have written for ten days of pills and a return visit they might not afford. Instead, he handed Sima a small strip of tablets and clear instructions: Three days. Come back if the fever rises or her breathing worsens, but three days should be enough.

Sima hesitated. Her sister in Jessore had told her that you must always finish a long course, that stopping early would only feed the germs. The doctor met her worry head-on. "We know more now," he said. For children like Amina with this level of pneumonia, a shorter course works just as well, and it is kinder to the body. He showed her how to mark each dose on the blister pack, then sent them home with a plan to return if she did not improve.

The first night was restless. By morning, the fever had drifted down. On day two, Amina asked for puffed rice with banana. On day three, she chased a stray chicken across the courtyard, laughing between small, leftover coughs.

The pills were gone, and the infection did not return.

Stories like hers are appearing from Dhaka to Denver. They tell the same truth. The old rule that long courses of antibiotics are always safer is not always right. For many common infections, shorter courses of treatment cure just as well, with fewer side effects and fewer chances for resistant bacteria to take root. It feels almost backward at first. We grew up with a single command printed on every bottle: Finish the entire course even if you feel better. That advice came from a place of fear and caution, and for a long time, it seemed beyond question.

To understand why this shift feels so radical, it helps to revisit where the long-course habit began. In the 1940s, penicillin, the first true antibiotic, had just been introduced. In his 1945 Nobel Prize speech, Sir Alexander Fleming, the discoverer of penicillin, gave a stern warning. He described a hypothetical patient who takes too little penicillin for a sore throat, not enough to kill the bacteria, just enough to teach them how to fight back. "If you use penicillin, use enough," Fleming cautioned. Doctors took this message to heart, interpreting it to mean that stopping antibiotics too early or using too low a dose could breed resistant germs. In those early days, with scant scientific data, physicians erred on the side of caution. They began prescribing antibiotics for fixed, lengthy durations—seven, ten, fourteen days or more—to ensure every last bacterium was wiped out. The intention was good: to protect patients from undertreatment. Over time, "finish the course" became virtually a sacred commandment in medicine.

For generations, this rule went unchallenged. Patients worldwide can recall a doctor's stern advice or a pharmacist's reminder sticker on the pill bottle: *Take all your pills even if you feel well.* In hospitals, protocols for infections were built around two-week or month-long courses as a standard. The idea of stopping early was almost heretical. Why risk it? No doctor wanted to be responsible for an infection flaring back up or a mutant germ emerging because treatment was cut short. As a result, in everything from ear infections to postsurgical wounds, longer antibiotic regimens became the default. It felt safe and reassuring, a bit like adding extra locks to a door after a break-in. More medicine meant more security, or so we all thought.

But as the years passed, cracks in this old belief started to appear. Ironically, while we worried so much about giving too few antibiotics, we overlooked the dangers of giving too much. Antibiotics, for all their lifesaving power, also carry serious collateral damage.

Patients on prolonged courses often suffer side effects, stomach pain, diarrhea, or stubborn yeast infections. Long courses can trigger the devastating *C. diff* infection we discussed in chapter 2. And the longer an antibiotic is given, the more it disrupts the body's healthy bacteria, and the more chances opportunistic, resistant bugs have to take over. In other words, using antibiotics for too long can sometimes create the very problems we feared. It is like flooding a garden to drown the weeds, only to find the floodwater invites a new infestation of pests.

By the 2000s, a few pioneering physicians and researchers began to ask uncomfortable questions. How long is long enough?

Could we maintain the same cure rates with a shorter treatment? These questions set the stage for a series of bold studies that would challenge medicine's prevailing wisdom. Initially, many in the medical community were skeptical, some were even angry, at the suggestion of cutting antibiotic courses. It went against everything they had been taught. But the only way to find the truth was to test it.

Evidence from the front lines

Over the last two decades, researchers have run hundreds of careful trials that put shorter antibiotic courses head to head with longer ones. Across many infections, the pattern is consistent. When care is done well, short courses cure as reliably as traditional regimens. Patients are no more likely to relapse, and they often do better because they avoid extra side effects, and fewer resistant bacteria are encouraged to grow.

One turning point was the STOP-IT trial. In 2015, surgeons and infectious disease teams across the United States asked a hard question about complicated intra-abdominal infections, the kind that follow a burst appendix or a drained abscess. Standard practice had been to prescribe eight to fourteen days of antibiotics after the source of infection was controlled. STOP-IT enrolled 518 patients and split them into two groups: those who received a fixed short course of four days after successful surgery or drainage, and those who received the traditional longer course that continued until fever and other signs had been gone for two days. The outcome was plain. About one in five patients in each group developed a post-treatment complication, and deaths were similar, at roughly 1%. The short-course patients were spared a week of drugs, with fewer opportunities for nausea, rashes, and resistance. Since then, guidelines have moved toward the simple rule the trial confirmed: Fix the source, then four days is enough.

Pneumonia told a similar story. In northern Spain, a study led by Dr. Ane Uranga treated hospitalized adults the usual way for the first few days, then reassessed on day five. If the fever had resolved and breathing had improved, antibiotics were stopped that day. Others continued on a longer course. Recovery at day ten was the same in both groups, and the short-course patients were less likely to be readmitted in the following month. Parallel trials in France and the Netherlands found that three to five days is often sufficient for mild to moderate cases once the patient turns the corner. Large studies in South Asia, including Bangladesh, showed that even three days can cure straightforward childhood pneumonia. The lesson is practical. When a patient is clearly better, continuing out of habit adds little benefit and more risk.

Urinary tract infections followed suit. For kidney infections in otherwise healthy women, Swedish investigators compared seven versus fourteen days of antibiotics. Cure rates were nearly identical, about 97% with the short course and 96% with the long. Side effects told the difference. Women on seven days had fewer problems, including fewer yeast infections, and they took half the total antibiotic exposure. For simple bladder infections, multiple trials have shown that three days usually works as well as a week. Shorter plans are also easier to finish, which means more patients take every prescribed dose correctly.

Consider the story of Poitr. He was forty-eight, the kind of man who could navigate Warsaw by sound alone. The squeal of the tram on Aleje Jerozolimskie. The hiss of buses at the Centrum stop. The winter air that smelled faintly of coal and exhaust and wet wool. He worked hard, kept his head down, and lately he'd been drinking more than he wanted to admit. At first, it was just to "take the edge off" after long days. Then it became the way he fell asleep.

In late January, Piotr caught the flu. The fever came fast, and the body aches even faster. He told himself it would pass, so he stayed home, sipped tea, and kept pouring vodka at night because it dulled the chills and quieted the cough. By day five, the flu was fading, but something else was moving in. His cough turned heavy and deep. He started breathing like he'd run up five flights of stairs, even while sitting still. When he finally walked into the emergency department, he was gray around the lips, sweating through his shirt, and trying to act tough even as his lungs did the opposite.

The chest X-ray confirmed pneumonia. His oxygen was low. They started antibiotics right away because this wasn't a "wait and see" moment. Then the blood cultures came back: Klebsiella in the bloodstream. That result changes the tone in a room. Pneumonia is serious. Pneumonia plus bacteria in the blood is the kind of serious that makes clinicians check your blood pressure twice and look at your kidneys, your heart rhythm, and your mental status. Piotr had risk stacked against him: influenza had inflamed his airways, heavy alcohol use had likely blunted his defenses and made aspiration more likely, and the infection had found a path from lung to blood.

But Piotr did something extraordinary: He responded quickly. Within two days, his fever broke. His blood pressure stabilized. His oxygen needs eased. The team watched him closely, repeated lab tests, and made sure the pneumonia was truly improving. This is the part most people don't realize: The goal isn't as many antibiotic days as possible. The goal is *enough days to cure the infection, and no more.*

For decades, doctors treated bloodstream infections like Piotr's as if fourteen days were a law of nature. Not because anyone proved two weeks was best, but because two weeks felt safe. The problem is that "safe" can quietly turn into "more than necessary," and antibiotics are not free. Every extra day increases the risk of diarrhea, nausea, yeast infections, drug reactions, and less visible harm: stripping the gut of protective bacteria and giving resistant germs more room to grow, a process you've already seen unfold in earlier chapters.

Researchers finally tested the habit. In one major study, patients who were clearly improving after a couple of days were assigned to either stop at seven days or continue to fourteen. The results were essentially the same. Another trial tried a slightly different approach: Some patients stopped based on a simple blood marker of inflammation (CRP), others stopped at seven days, and others went the full fourteen. Again, the shorter approaches held up just as well in straightforward cases. A third trial in similar bloodstream infections reached the same conclusion: When the source is controlled, and the patient is truly turning the corner, seven days can be enough.

That's why Piotr's doctors didn't cut his treatment short. They finished it. They treated the infection hard up front, watched for real improvement, and then stopped when the job was done. One less week of antibiotics meant fewer side effects and less collateral damage, without sacrificing safety. The point isn't to ration care. It's to replace autopilot medicine with the kind that's precise: the right drug, for the right patient, for the right length of time.

Here's the plain-language version: Imagine you've always been told that the best way to get home is driving fourteen miles by winding back roads. Then someone points out there's a seven-mile highway—straight, clear, and faster. These studies asked: *If the highway is open and conditions are right, why take the long route?* In those cases, the seven-mile trip was just as safe.

Piotr went home breathing easier, weaker than he expected, but alive and improving. Before he left, one of the doctors said something simple: "The antibiotics did their job. Now we have to let *your body* do the rest." In modern medicine, that sentence is easy to forget.

And if Piotr's story feels uncomfortably familiar to anyone reading in Warsaw or anywhere else, that's the point. The science is global, but the lesson is personal: Sometimes the safest antibiotic plan is not the longest one, but the *right-length* one.

Taken together, these trials do not say "short for everything." They say, "short" when the source is controlled, the diagnosis is clear, and the patient is improving. That is a careful kind of medicine. It is also kinder. Fewer days mean fewer harms, less disruption of the microbiome, and less fuel for resistance, while delivering the same chance of cure.

A Global Movement Takes Hold

The wins in abdominal infections, pneumonia, bacteremia, and UTIs did more than change a few protocols. They lit a fuse. What began as quiet debates in journal clubs has grown into a worldwide shift in how we think about antibiotics. Guideline writers took notice. In the United States and across Europe, pneumonia recommendations were updated to say that three to five days is often enough once a patient stabilizes. Surgical societies began to endorse short, fixed courses after the source of an abdominal infection was controlled. In primary care, the reflex to hand out a week of pills for every cough softened, with clearer advice to skip antibiotics for viral illness and to shorten courses when bacterial disease is confirmed.

Change is happening far from academic hospitals, too. In Lima, a public hospital that once sent women home with an "extra week just in case" after kidney infections audited its outcomes. After adopting seven days as the default, return visits did not rise, and patients reported fewer side effects. Clinics in Southeast Asia and sub-Saharan Africa have run similar checks, trimming days where the evidence supports it and finding the same thing: Patients do just as well, and often feel better, when we stop sooner.

Perhaps the most encouraging shift is in the conversation between clinicians and patients. The old command to "finish everything, no matter what" is giving way to a plan with checkpoints. Doctors explain up front why a shorter course is being used, what improvement to look for by day three or day five, and when to call if things stall. Patients, in turn, share how they are feeling and help decide whether to continue or stop. When a longer course truly is needed, the reason is made clear. This partnership builds trust, improves adherence, and keeps treatment tailored to the person, not to tradition.

When less becomes more

It is natural to wonder how fewer pills can heal as well as more. The answer lives in the biology of infection. In many common illnesses, antibiotics deliver most of their benefit in the first few days, knocking the bacterial load down to a level the immune system can handle. Once fever has settled and breathing, pain, or urination are back on track, continuing the drug rarely adds protection. What it does add is risk: more nausea and rashes, more *C. diff* in vulnerable patients, and more pressure on your microbiome that can favor resistant strains. So, there is a sweet spot: Treat just long enough to help the body overcome the infection, then stop. Overshooting that mark does not improve the outcome; it just tilts the risk-benefit balance in the wrong direction.

Think of a campfire that is already out. One bucket of water does the job. A second and third bucket do not make it "more out," they only soak the ground and wash away good soil. Antibiotics work the same way. Once the flames are gone, extra buckets bring harm without benefit. Stopping once the fire is out is common sense. For years, medicine kept pouring, just to be sure. Now we know when enough is enough.

Shorter does not mean short for everything. Some infections, like tuberculosis or certain bone and heart infections, still demand long courses. The shift is not about cutting corners, it is about right-sizing. We test, we measure, and we stop when the data and the patient's recovery say it is time.

In practice, the benefits of this shift are far-reaching. For individual patients, it means fewer days tied to pill schedules or IV lines, fewer drug-related complications, and faster return to daily life. For healthcare systems, it means reduced costs, shorter hospital stays, fewer prescriptions filled, and less burden from the complications of antibiotic overuse.

And on a global scale, using antibiotics more judiciously buys us crucial time in the war against antibiotic resistance. Superbugs thrive on our excesses. Every unnecessary dose is like giving the enemy ammunition. By cutting out those excesses, we disarm the enemy little by little. One large study even found that patients who received excessively long courses for abdominal infections were more likely to develop new resistant infections and had higher mortality. Overtreating can be as dangerous as undertreating, a lesson we are finally beginning to heed.

Cost saving in action.

At a midsize hospital in the Midwest, a small change quietly reshaped care. The pneumonia order set had always defaulted to seven days of antibiotics. No one argued with it because that was how things were done. Then a pilot program tried something different. If a patient with uncomplicated community-acquired pneumonia met clear stability criteria by day three to five, the team stopped antibiotics at day five, and sometimes at day three. The shift felt modest, almost shy, yet the ripple effects were hard to miss.

Patients noticed first. They went home sooner, with fewer pills and fewer side effects. Nurses saw it next. With shorter courses and earlier discharge, they reclaimed hours that had been swallowed by routine medication passes and monitoring. Physicians had more time for complex patients who truly needed it. The building itself seemed to breathe easier. Freeing half a day to nearly a day of hospitalization per case opened dozens of bed-days across a hundred admissions, the equivalent of creating capacity without adding a single room.

The numbers told the same story. Each patient who moved from a seven-day plan to five saved the hospital a meaningful sum in direct costs and freed several hours of nursing and physician time. When the course stopped at three days for the simplest cases, the savings were even larger, along with a full shift of nursing time returned to the unit. Stretch that across a year's worth of admissions and you are looking at hundreds of bed-days recovered, well over a million dollars in avoided costs, and thousands of clinical hours redirected to higher-value care. Even patients' wallets felt the difference, with fewer out-of-pocket prescriptions to fill at discharge.

None of this required heroics. The team added a day-three checklist, flipped to oral antibiotics early, and built an automatic stop unless the clinician chose to continue for a clear reason. Readmissions did not rise. Outcomes did not worsen. In fact, patients often felt better faster, likely because their bodies were spared unnecessary days of medication.

This is what "less is more" looks like when it leaves the page and lands on a ward. Shorter courses, when a patient is stable, do not cut corners. They trim waste. They protect patients from harm we used to accept as the cost of being thorough. They give time back to nurses and doctors who never seem to have enough of it. And they keep beds open for the next person who needs one. In a world where antibiotics are losing ground, doing only what is necessary is not just prudent medicine; it is a lifeline for patients and hospitals alike.

A new mindset and hope for the future

The move to shorter antibiotic courses is not a tweak; it is a change in how we think. It asks clinicians to trade habit for evidence, to treat precisely rather than generously, and to invite patients into the plan. Less can be an act of wisdom. It takes humility to set aside the reflex to be "safe" with extra days, and it takes trust to stop when the job is done. This shift has been slow to build, study by study and bedside by bedside, but the momentum is real.

The reward is tangible. Fewer pills mean fewer side effects, steadier stomachs, and less risk of dangerous complications like *C. diff.* Families spend less on prescriptions. Hospitals see beds open sooner. Most importantly, patients feel better faster because their bodies are not dragged through unnecessary treatment. Picture a child in Dhaka who needs only five days instead of ten, or a grandfather in Ohio who avoids a second illness because his course ends at day five. These are small victories that add up to healthier lives.

There is a more profound lesson underneath. Medicine evolves. What felt like gospel yesterday can be tested today and improved tomorrow. "Finish the course no matter what" sounded safe for decades. Now we know that right-sized care is safer. Five days when a patient is stable. More only when the science says it is needed. Every time we choose the minimum effective dose, we protect the person in front of us and we protect the power of antibiotics for the person who will need them next year.

This way of thinking does not end with antibiotics. It nudges us to ask, in every corner of care, how little is enough. Fewer days on an IV. Fewer scans when reassurance will do. Fewer interventions that add cost and risk without adding benefit. The goal is not to do less for its own sake. The goal is to do exactly what works.

Which raises a final question. If the safest antibiotic is the one you do not take, what would it look like to prevent more infections in the first place? Clean hands. Clean water. Vaccines. Smarter hospital design. Community habits that reduce the likelihood of illness.

That is where this story goes next. In the following chapter, "Preventing Infections," we will explore proactive measures that stop infections and outbreaks before they begin. We will meet the people and ideas that stop outbreaks before they start, spare patients the ordeal of treatment, and keep our best medicines in reserve for when they are truly needed. The idea of "less is more" begins with shorter courses, but its most significant potential is realized when no treatment is needed at all.

Key ideas

- Short, targeted therapy often works as well as longer courses, with fewer harms.
- Reassessment is a feature, not a failure.

Do this — Readers

- Ask about the shortest effective course and whether watchful waiting is safe.
- Be open to "stop early if better" plans your clinician suggests.

Do this — Clinicians

- Cite the evidence for short courses; build stop dates into orders.
- Normalize "antibiotic time-out" language with teams and patients.
- Use delayed prescriptions and safety-netting where appropriate.

Conversation starters

- "What is the shortest course demonstrated to work for this?"
- "How will we follow up if we try watchful waiting?"

Chapter 11

Preventing Infections

At 3 a.m. in West Hartford, Connecticut, the streetlights along Farmington Avenue glowed on wet pavement after a passing shower. Alina lay curled beneath a thin quilt, counting the seconds to the next stab of pain in her lower abdomen. Every few minutes, she shuffled down the narrow hallway of her apartment to the bathroom, whispering a weary prayer that the burning would ease: another urinary tract infection, her second in three months. The city felt hushed. Only the hum of the fridge and the whoosh of an occasional car on I-84 kept her company.

She replayed the past day like a film. A long train ride back from Stamford with hardly a sip of water. Two meetings in New Haven, where she ignored the need to pee. A late dinner, then straight to bed. In the medicine cabinet, the half-finished antibiotics from last time stared back at her. She shut the door gently. Her doctor had been clear: Get tested, use the right antibiotic only if needed, and take it exactly as prescribed. No guessing, no leftovers.

At dawn, she drove to an urgent care near Blue Back Square. The ritual unfolded as always: a cup, a sample, a careful history. The clinician listened, kind but direct. "UTIs are common, especially in women. We can treat this. Let's also keep it from coming back." Alina felt a knot loosen. She was tired of reacting. She wanted a plan.

Back home, she started small and steady. A big glass of water with breakfast, then a refill before lunch, then again midafternoon. She set a gentle reminder on her phone to take bathroom breaks, even on busy days. In the bathroom, she kept it simple, front to back when wiping, no harsh soaps, just warm water. She switched to breathable underwear and avoided staying in workout clothes after a run on the Farmington Canal trail. With her partner, she added two easy habits: pee before and after sex, wash gently, no douching, no spermicides. None of it felt dramatic. All of it felt doable.

She asked about cranberries. The clinician explained it this way: Some cranberry products can help certain women by making it harder for bacteria to stick to the bladder wall. If she wanted to try, she should choose an unsweetened juice or a standardized capsule and keep expectations realistic. They talked through other options, too. For now, no daily antibiotics, save that tool for later if needed. If UTIs returned often, they would check for triggers, review contraception, and consider additional strategies. The point was to prevent, not chase.

Weeks slipped by. The maple trees along Fern Street turned from lime to emerald. Alina kept a water bottle in her tote and a spare in the car. She stopped holding it during meetings. She learned to recognize early bladder whispers and to answer them. A month passed without a flare. Then two. Then three. The fear that had shadowed her mornings began to fade. When friends gathered on her porch for iced tea in late September, she told them what had helped. Not a miracle pill. Just a handful of consistent habits and a promise to herself to act early rather than endure.

Prevention is not only personal. It is the air we share, the water we drink, and the care we give one another. Bathing is part routine, part quiet maintenance of your body's first shield. A quick shower after workouts, gardening, or a long commute rinses away sweat, soil, and the film that microbes love. Gentle soap, warm water, and a soft towel are enough.

Harsh scrubs and scalding water strip the skin, leaving it dry and cracked. After you wash, a light, unscented moisturizer keeps that barrier supple so tiny fissures do not become doorways. Think of it as daily upkeep, like oiling a hinge. Small care, fewer openings, fewer infections.

Bedding carries our hours with it. Skin cells, oils, and the germs we collect during the day settle into sheets and pillowcases. Wash sheets weekly in warm or hot water. Change pillowcases more often if you are sick, if you wear hair products to bed, or if you are prone to skin breakouts. Towels do their best work when they are clean and dry, so swap them every few uses and let them hang open between showers. If a stomach bug or a respiratory virus moves through the house, give linens a fresh cycle, run bath mats and gym clothes through the wash, and let everything dry thoroughly. A simple rhythm of bathing and clean bedding turns nights of rest into quiet prevention.

In the quiet before dawn at a busy city hospital, Dr. Arun jogged from one room to the next after an eighteen-hour shift. A monitor alarm chirped. He ducked into a restroom and splashed water on his face. As his hand moved toward the soap dispenser… A pager buzzed. He hesitated, then hurried toward a postoperative patient. Days later, that patient spiked a fever. Cultures grew a bacterium often carried on hands. No one could pinpoint the exact moment of transmission, yet the lesson landed with a thud. Dr. Arun stood at the bedside and made a quiet promise. *No more shortcuts. Alcohol rub at the door. Soap and water when soiled. Every time, every room.*

That promise is the heart of this chapter. Antibiotics rescue us after the spark has caught. Prevention keeps the spark from landing. For Alina, prevention looked like water on the desk, a bathroom break on time, and a short list of gentle routines.

For a hospital, it is clean hands, early catheter removal, and tight lines on cleaning and device care. For a neighborhood, it is safe drinking water, working toilets, and vaccines that stop infections before they start. These are not grand gestures. They are ordinary acts done on time, over and over, until they change the story.

The pages ahead are a practical field guide. We will start at home with habits that lower the odds of common infections. We will step into clinics and wards to see how design, check-lists, and culture make prevention visible and easy. We will widen the lens to communities, where clean water, sanitation, and vaccination save more lives than any pill ever could. The goal is simple: fewer infections to treat, fewer antibiotics to take, and stronger medicines when we truly need them.

Alina's year did not turn on a single decision. It turned on many small ones, stacked like bricks, steady and unremark-able. That is how prevention works. Quietly at first. Then all at once.

Handwashing: The First Line of Defense

The morning after his patient's fever broke, Dr. Arun stood at the sink outside the ICU and watched the water run. He could still hear the man's question in his head: *How did this happen to me?* The answer was ordinary, which made it heavy. He had rushed, skipped the sink for a few seconds, then touched a chart, a rail, a wound dressing. One shortcut, one chain of touches, one infection that never needed to happen.

That week, the hospital took a hard look at itself. A quiet audit showed what busy places often reveal: excellent peo-ple, imperfect habits. Hand rubs were empty at a few doors. Sinks were tucked behind carts. Posters were faded and easy to ignore. No one meant harm. There was simply no margin in crowded hallways and long shifts. So they moved dispensers to the places where hands actually pause. They added bright, simple signs at eye level. They started a norm that anyone could offer a friendly nudge, a nurse to doctor, a patient to phlebotomist: "Clean in, clean out?" Dr. Arun began modeling it without fuss, using soap and water before and after every patient, using alcohol rub when moving fast, and using a complete wash after the restroom. Within months, the small things added up. Line infections dropped. Surgical sites healed without drama. Families noticed. "Doctor, did you clean your hands?" became a welcome question.

Handwashing sounds like kindergarten advice. It is also one of the most powerful interventions in modern medicine. The gap is not knowledge; it is consistency. People forget. People hurry. Yet microbes never do. They move from skin to surface to skin in seconds, especially after the bathroom, after blowing a nose, after touching a phone that has been everywhere. You cannot see the transfer, but the patient with a fresh incision will feel its consequences.

The power of clean hands isn't just a hospital story; it's a global story. In many parts of the world, the fight for hand hygiene is a fight for basic resources. Picture a small village clinic in a rural area where water is scarce. A midwife named Amina recalls how, years ago, new mothers and babies in her community often fell ill with fevers after childbirth. With a limited understanding of germs, they didn't realize that the traditional practice of delivering babies with unwashed hands was contributing to deadly infections. Amina herself lost a baby early in her career, a heartbreaking loss that local custom attributed to fate. But Amina suspected there was something more at play. Determined to honor that baby's memory, she sought training and learned about infection prevention.

Armed with new knowledge, she returned to her village with a mission: to make handwashing a ritual as sacred as the birth itself. She worked to secure a simple handwashing station, a bucket with a tap, clean water, and soap in the dirt-floored birthing room. At first, the older midwives were skeptical, but Amina gently insisted, telling the story of the child who we now know likely died of a preventable infection. Over time, her colleagues embraced the change. They scrubbed up to their elbows before each delivery and again afterward. The effect was extraordinary. The rates of fever and infection in mothers and newborns plummeted. Word spread to neighboring villages, and soon more clinics adopted "Amina's clean hands" practice. What was once viewed as unnecessary began to be seen as an act of love and professionalism.

If the last few years taught us anything, it is that habits scale. During the pandemic, the world learned to hum a song while scrubbing. Then, as fear faded, so did the habit. The lesson remains. You will rarely know which wash prevented which infection. You will only see calmer wards, fewer prescriptions, fewer grandparents in ICU beds, and more newborns going home without a fever.

We pass germs along with what we touch most, and nothing gets more mileage than a phone. It rides in bathrooms, on cafeteria tables, on bus seats, and then rests against our cheeks. Make a quiet rule: wash or sanitize your hands, then clean the phone. A simple microfiber cloth most days, and a 70% isopropyl alcohol wipe on high-exposure days, is enough for most devices. Pop the case off once a week and wipe the edges and buttons. Do the same for shared tablets and workstations. Clean hands matter. So do the things our clean hands touch next.

Fingernails are tiny shelves where bacteria love to linger. Keep them short enough that you can see the skin of the fingertip, not the nail past it. Scrub under nails when you wash, especially after the bathroom, gardening, cooking, or a commute. Skip artificial nails if you work with patients or prepare food; they trap moisture and make hand hygiene less effective. Avoid cutting your cuticles too deeply. Just nudge them back after a shower and keep the skin moisturized so it doesn't crack. Small care, big payoff.

Outside hospitals, the same rhythm protects families. Wash before cooking, before eating, after the bathroom, after changing diapers, after handling trash or pet waste, and when you come home from crowded places. In schools and offices, put sanitizer where hands naturally reach, at classroom doors, near elevators, beside conference tables. Make it easy to do the right thing without thinking.

Coughs and sneezes are how many infections hitch a ride. Make it a routine to cover your mouth and nose with a tissue, then throw it away and clean your hands. No tissue handy? Tuck the cough into your elbow, not your palm. This keeps droplets off the doorknobs, phones, and railings that everyone shares. If you are under the weather, a well-fitted mask in crowded indoor spaces is a courtesy that protects the very young, the very old, and anyone whose immune system is working overtime.

There is another quiet habit that matters more than most of us admit. Our hands visit our faces dozens of times an hour. Rubbing tired eyes, biting a nail, or picking the nose is a straight path for germs to the places they like best. Keep nails short and smooth so they are easier to clean and less likely to harbor grime. Make "hands off the face" a family cue. Teachers use it, nurses use it, and it works at home, too. Pair that with a pocket pack of tissues, a small hand sanitizer, good ventilation, a cracked window, a kitchen fan, a few minutes of fresh air between visitors, and you have a simple respiratory toolkit that keeps coughs from becoming chains of infection.

If a cold or flu moves through the house, turn these habits up a notch. Set a small "tissue and trash" station where people gather, wipe high-touch surfaces daily, and remind each other with a smile rather than a scold. Little practices, done consistently, keep microbes from leaping hand to hand and face to face.

So what does proper handwashing actually mean? It means using clean water and soap to scrub every surface of the hands, palms, backs, between fingers, under nails, for about twenty seconds (roughly the time it takes to hum a couple of verses of your favorite song). It means doing it every time it matters: before eating or cooking, after using the bathroom, after caring for someone sick or tending to a wound, after handling garbage or dirty diapers, and whenever your hands are visibly dirty. In healthcare settings, it means before and after every patient contact, and, yes, absolutely before and after using the restroom, even if you're a busy doctor or nurse. For those moments when soap and water aren't available, alcohol-based hand sanitizers are a good replacement, but nothing beats a thorough hand wash if you can do it. It may feel mundane, but think of it this way: Each time you wash your hands, you're potentially breaking a chain of infection. You're stopping a microscopic foe from traveling from your hands to someone's vulnerable body.

Handwashing truly deserves to be called "the world's oldest new medicine." It's old wisdom: The Bible, the Quran, and other ancient texts reference ritual handwashing. It took until the nineteenth century for science to catch up, when Dr. Ignaz Semmelweis famously demonstrated that doctors with clean hands saved mothers from deadly childbed fever.

Sadly, Semmelweis's colleagues in 1840s Vienna resisted his findings, and it took decades for handwashing to be universally adopted. Today, we have no excuse. We know the science, and we've heard the stories. The challenge isn't knowledge anymore; it's consistency and commitment. But every person can rise to that challenge.

Skin and Wound Care: Protecting the Body's Barrier

On a bright June morning in Toronto, the peonies along Gladys's back fence were finally in full bloom. She put on her straw hat, slipped into her old canvas sneakers, and stepped onto the small patch of lawn behind her semi-detached home in Leslieville. The sound of a streetcar bell ringing from Queen Street drifted over the fences, and a gull called from somewhere near the lake. Gladys, a retired grade 3 teacher, knelt down to prune a stubborn rose cane that had strayed where it shouldn't be.

She felt a prick at her ankle before she saw it, a quick sting followed by a bead of blood, but then the pain diminished. She rinsed the area with the hose, dabbed it with the corner of her T-shirt, and reminded herself not to fuss. She had a trip to the farmers market at Withrow Park to make, and later, her grandkids were coming over for popsicles on the porch. Toronto summers are short, and she wasn't going to waste one on a little scratch.

Two days later, the nick had not scabbed. By the third, her ankle felt hot in her sock, and the skin around the cut was flushed. Still, she kept moving, hopping the TTC to her line dancing class at the community center, telling herself it would settle. When the pain began climbing toward her calf and a fever crept in, her daughter found her on the couch, pale and sweating, a bag of frozen peas pressed to her leg. They headed for the emergency department at Michael Garron, inching along the Gardiner Expressway, a ribbon of brake lights out the window as the city sweltered.

The diagnosis was blunt. A common skin bacterium, likely *Staphylococcus* aureus from the garden soil or even from her own skin, had slipped through that tiny break and was now racing through the tissues of her lower leg. The doctor added a piece of news that made the room go quiet. Gladys's blood sugar was high. Undiagnosed diabetes had been quietly narrowing blood vessels and blunting her immune response. What should have been a small, fussy wound had found the perfect opening.

Intravenous antibiotics were started within an hour. Nurses wrapped her leg, lifted it on pillows, and checked her temperature through the night. The pain softened, then flared again. An ultrasound showed sluggish flow in a few vessels. A vascular team performed a procedure to improve circulation. The big words that had scared her on day one, *sepsis* and *amputation*, faded from the conversation. Three weeks later, the swelling had eased, the skin looked calmer, and the wound finally knit in from the edges. She went home with a cane, a new glucose meter, and a healthy respect for what her skin does for her every day.

Back in her garden by August, Gladys had new rules. Proper boots and gloves. No more bare-ankle weeding. If she nicked herself, she washed the area right away with tap water and a little mild soap, patted it dry, and covered it with a clean bandage from the drawer near the kettle. No hydrogen peroxide this time. She learned that it can be harsh on healthy skin cells and may slow healing. Each evening, she checked the spot under good light and changed the dressing. Any spreading redness, warmth, thick discharge, fever, or pain that felt worse rather than better meant she would call her family doctor. She also learned a winter lesson that matters in Toronto's dry, radiator season. Dry, cracked skin is full of tiny doorways for germs. A simple unscented moisturizer after a shower helps keep the barrier intact. It is comfort, yes, but it is also prevention.

Her diabetes diagnosis reshaped the small things, too. She met with a diabetes educator at the clinic, adjusted her diet without giving up her Sunday bagel, and added a short loop through Riverdale Park to her morning walk. Most importantly, she built a habit that every Torontonian with diabetes is urged to keep. Daily foot checks. A quick look between toes and along heels to catch blisters, hot spots, or cuts early, especially if sensation is dulled. If something looked off, she did not wait.

Gladys's close call carries a simple truth. Skin is your castle wall. When it is intact, it turns away the countless microbes you meet on door handles, subway poles, garden soil, and pet fur. When there is a breach, even a pinprick, bacteria can take their chance. Most of the time your body handles it just fine. A clot forms, a scab seals, and the immune system does its quiet work. But if circulation is poor, if the immune system is tired, or if the bacteria are particularly aggressive, a small opening can become a big problem fast. The rare, headline-grabbing horrors like necrotizing soft tissue infection often start exactly this way, from an ordinary cut that becomes contaminated and is missed until pain and swelling explode. The lesson is not to panic. It is to act early and simply.

Good wound care is first aid, and it is also stewardship. Clean water to flush out grit. Gentle soap if it is dirty. A clean dressing to keep new dirt out. Watchful eyes over the following days. Seek help if it is getting worse instead of better. Those few minutes at the sink can spare you a course of antibiotics, a clinic visit, and a week of worry. Wound care starts before the bandage. Short, clean nails make cleaning easier and keep new germs out. If you nick yourself while cooking or gardening, rinse the cut, wash your hands, then give the nail edges a quick scrub so debris doesn't sneak back in when you re-dress the wound. It takes a minute and lowers the odds you'll be back for antibiotics later. Scale that across a city of gardeners, cyclists, cooks, and kids, and you see the broader effect. Each infection prevented is one less reason to reach for antibiotics, one less nudge toward resistance.

There is an emotional piece here as well. People are often surprised that a small cut can lead to significant consequences; they feel fear when a fever hits, and sometimes guilt for "not taking it seriously." Be kind to yourself and be practical. Clean the wound. Cover it. Check it. Care for your skin, especially in seasons when the air is dry and hands are washed often. If you live with conditions like eczema or diabetes, give your skin a little extra attention and plan foot checks into the day the way you plan your Presto reloads or your coffee runs.

These are small, local habits, the kind that fit into a Toronto morning without fuss. They are also universal. Whether you are pruning roses in Leslieville, walking the boardwalk at the Beaches, or teaching a child in Accra how to clean a scraped knee, the steps are the same. Our skin protects us quietly. When it needs help, give it quickly.

Vaccination: Our Collective Shield

On a humid evening in Orlando, the cicadas were loud enough to feel like a soundtrack. Chelsey stood by the crib in her townhouse near Lake Eola, rocking her five-month-old, Kaliah, through another restless night. It had started as a runny nose, the kind you chalk up to daycare germs or Florida pollen. By day three, a fever arrived. Then a scatter of tiny red spots on her hairline that crept down behind her ears. Kaliah grew fussier, her eyes watery, her breathing a little faster than usual. Chelsey had seen news about measles popping up in Florida, but it felt far away, like a storm spinning offshore.

In the pediatric ER, the triage nurse's tone shifted when she heard "fever, rash, red eyes." A swab, a room with the door closed, a mask on, and then a pediatrician who pulled a chair close and spoke gently. It looked like measles. The tests would confirm it, but everything fit. Kaliah was admitted for fluids and close monitoring. For three days, Chelsey sat by the crib, listening to the soft whoosh of oxygen, watching the parade of gloved hands and careful eyes. The rash marched down Kaliah's arms and belly. Her fever climbed, then broke. When the lab results came back, the doctor nodded. Positive.

Chelsey's heart sank. She is not careless or unloving. She is a Florida mom doing her best, juggling a return to work, a tight budget, and a swirl of advice from family, social media, and friends. She and her husband had planned to start Kaliah's routine shots right on schedule, but measles protection comes later, usually at twelve to fifteen months. Infants that young rely on the immunity of the people around them. In the weeks before Kaliah got sick, Chelsey had skipped a church potluck when she heard about an outbreak two counties over. She wiped grocery cart handles at Publix. She did most of the things any parent would do. What she didn't know was that a single contagious person in a crowded indoor space can leave the virus hanging in the air for hours. You can walk in after they've left and still get sick. Measles is that contagious.

The guilt came like a rip current. *Did I miss something? Did I put her at risk?* The team stayed with her in that moment.

They explained what many Floridians are now relearning. Measles travels fast and far, especially when vaccination rates dip. No one choice caused this, and she was not alone. The path forward was care and recovery, then learning how to build the strongest shield for her family.

Kaliah recovered, and within a week the rash faded to a memory. Chelsey went home with relief and with a deeper understanding of what vaccines actually do. They are not only an individual seat belt, but they are also a community guardrail. When enough of us are immune, a virus like measles runs out of road. It bumps into person after person who cannot catch it, and the chain of transmission snaps. That is how we protect babies like Kaliah, who are too young for their own measles shot. That is how we protect a neighbor on chemotherapy in Tampa, or a grandfather with a lung condition in Jacksonville, or the teacher in Gainesville who takes immunosuppressing medicines for arthritis.

If you live in Florida, this is not abstract. Theme parks draw families from every corner of the globe. Cruise ports hum. Airports move millions. Ball games, church services, indoor play spaces on steamy afternoons, shelters during hurricane season, all put us shoulder to shoulder. That is part of the beauty of life here, and part of why community immunity matters so much. Measles needs only a tiny gap to return.

To smother it, coverage needs to be very high, typically around 95% with the two-dose MMR series.

Talking about vaccines can be hard. People have questions, and that is reasonable. Some worry about side effects or feel overwhelmed by the schedule. Others were raised on mixed messages or know a friend of a friend with a scary story. If that is you, you deserve straight answers without judgment. Here is what helps many parents feel steadier.

First, measles is not a mild rite of passage. It can lead to pneumonia, dehydration, ear infections that cause hearing loss, and, rarely, brain swelling that can be fatal. Even in well-resourced hospitals, clinicians hold their breath when a very young infant or a child with other health issues gets measles.

Second, the MMR vaccine has been used for decades and has been studied more than almost any other medical intervention. Serious reactions are very rare. Fever and a brief rash can occur. Severe allergic reactions are uncommon. The benefits, for most children, far outweigh those short-lived risks.

Third, timing matters. Most children get MMR at twelve to fifteen months, then a booster at four to six years, often required for kindergarten entry. During outbreaks or before international travel, babies six to eleven months can receive an early extra dose to bridge that vulnerable period. Adults who are unsure whether they were vaccinated can get a simple blood test or a dose to catch up. If you have questions about your own history, ask your doctor or your county health department. They answer these questions every day.

The idea is not to shame anyone into a corner. It is to build a circle. In recent Florida outbreaks, communities have responded with practical kindness. Pediatric offices opened Saturday clinics. County vans parked at libraries and church lots on hot afternoons, offering MMR to anyone who needed it. Pharmacists at Publix and CVS rolled up sleeves between flu shots and blood pressure checks. Parents shared rides, watched each other's kids, and passed along accurate information. When enough people stepped in, transmission chains fizzled out.

Chelsey sometimes thinks back to the moment a nurse handed her a bottle of water and sat down, unhurried, to answer every question. That posture—calm, present, respectful—changed everything. It turned fear into action. She finished Kaliah's routine vaccines on schedule, talked with her own parents about boosters before holiday gatherings, and encouraged friends to ask their pediatricians the same questions she had asked. Not lecturing, just sharing what she had learned the hard way.

If you are on the fence, here are a few practical steps, offered in that same spirit.

- Check your family's vaccine records. If anything is missing, make a plan with your clinician. In Florida, many pharmacies can vaccinate older children and adults, often without a long wait.

- Ask your pediatrician about an early MMR dose if you have a baby under one year during an outbreak.

- Confirm that everyone is up to date before travel, especially international trips or cruises.

- Let your circle know if you or a loved one cannot be vaccinated for medical reasons. Friends can surround you with their immunity.

Vaccination rarely feels heroic in the moment. It is a quiet appointment squeezed between school pick-up and a grocery run. A tiny sting and a sticker. Yet multiplied across neighborhoods from Pensacola to Fort Lauderdale, those tiny acts add up to something profound.

They keep newborns out of hospital cribs. They keep schools open and grandparents' hugs safe. They give doctors space to fight the infections we cannot prevent.

Measles is a test of how much we are willing to look out for one another. Florida knows how to do that. They board up windows together in storm season, share generators, and check on neighbors. Building a shield of immunity around our most vulnerable is the same kind of care, just quieter. If you have questions, ask them. If you are ready, roll up a sleeve.

Chelsey will tell you it is not about winning an argument. It is about the baby sleeping in the next room, and the one down the block, and the ones we will welcome into this sun-soaked state tomorrow.

Hope, Responsibility, and the Power of Simple Habits

All through this chapter, we have walked beside people whose lives bent at quiet crossroads. A doctor pausing at a sink. A mother reaching for a soap dispenser in a village clinic. A grandmother taking a nick on her ankle seriously. A parent choosing a vaccine in a crowded waiting room. Different places, different stakes, the same lesson. It is far better to prevent an infection than to fight it once it takes hold. That is not just a medical principle; it is a human one. Prevention gives us time, preserves our strength, and keeps families together.

Think of what happens when simple habits take root. Handwashing cuts chains of transmission that would otherwise run through a school, a workplace, or a ward. In communities that teach and support regular hand hygiene, children miss fewer days of class, postoperative fevers fall, and stomach bugs lose momentum. A bar of soap and twenty seconds of attention can change a season for an entire neighborhood. The same is true for careful skin and wound care. Clean water over a scrape, a clean dressing, a daily glance for early redness, and a timely visit if pain rises. That small pattern prevents unnecessary emergency surgeries and spares antibiotics for when they are truly needed.

Vaccination sits alongside those habits as a shared shield. One appointment protects the person in the chair and the people they love. It protects the newborn who is too young for shots, the neighbor on chemotherapy, and the teacher whose immune system is fragile. The science here is steady and clear, yet what moves people is not a chart. It is the memory of a child's cough that eased because a virus never arrived, the relief of a healthy checkup after a season of outbreaks, the quiet knowledge that your choice helped keep someone else safe.

Underneath the science is something more ordinary and more powerful. It is the daily willingness to try. A nurse who sanitizes before every room, even at midnight. A father who keeps a small bottle of alcohol hand sanitizer in the car and makes handwashing part of the return-home routine. A teenager who asks for her vaccine record because she wants to be up to date before travel. These are modest acts, repeated by millions, that add up to fewer funerals and more ordinary days. In public health, we talk about "population impact." In real life, it feels like a grandmother at a birthday party instead of a hospital bed, and a parent at a school concert instead of an urgent care.

Prevention also buys us something precious that rarely makes headlines. It buys time. Every infection that never happens is one less course of antibiotics given. That is one less roll of the dice for resistance, one more day that a last-resort drug will still work for a stranger we will never meet. In that sense, washing your hands or bandaging a cut is not only self-care. It is stewardship. It says, *I will use this era's medical gifts wisely so they remain gifts for those who come after me.*

None of this is about perfection. People forget. Water runs cold in winter. Life gets busy and weary and loud. What matters is not flawless practice, but faithful practice. You will miss a step sometimes. Start again at the next sink. Replace the box of bandages on the kitchen shelf. Schedule the next dose on your way out of the clinic. Small resets keep the habits alive.

And there is a ripple effect. A child watches a parent scrub palms, backs of hands, between fingers, under nails, and grows up doing it without thinking. A patient asks, kindly, "Would you sanitize first?" and a nurse smiles and says, *Thank you*. A coach keeps sanitizer on the sideline, and a classroom keeps tissues and a bin by the door. A temple, or church, or mosque posts a reminder near the restroom, and a café adds a hand-washing sign near the sink. The idea travels faster than the microbes do because people talk, imitate, and care.

It helps to remember what prevention is not. It is not a scold. It is not a contest to see who is purest or bravest. It is a community pact. We look out for one another in ways that are visible and invisible. On the days when your habits protect me, I may never know it. On the days when mine protect you, you may never know it, either. That is the beauty of this work. It is shared, and it is generous. Tiny habits travel far: Clean your hands, clean your phone, keep nails short and healthy, and you've just broken three links in a chain of infection.

We have walked through the body's quiet rooms together. A liver that tried to filter a cure and ended up injured by it. A gut that lost its familiar rhythm after a routine course and could not find its way back quickly. A kidney that held the line until it didn't, and turned an ordinary infection into a longer, harder recovery. Different organs, different stories, but the same lesson: Antibiotics are not just something we take. They are something we steward. The goal has never been to use them less for the sake of using them less. It has been to use them well enough that the help they offer doesn't come with needless harm. And prevention is where that stewardship starts.

So let this be the charge we carry forward. Wash your hands with intention. Tend every cut as if it matters, because it does. Keep skin healthy so the body's first barrier stays strong. Stay current on vaccines, and ask questions until you feel informed and respected. If you are a clinician, make prevention visible and easy for patients. If you lead a school, a team, or a faith community, build these habits into the way your group cares for one another. If you make policy, remember that clean water, good ventilation, safe staffing, and access to vaccines are not luxuries. They are the infrastructure of everyday health.

Imagine where this takes us. A ward where fewer patients need isolation because infections do not spread in the first place. A clinic where parents sit quietly with healthy infants during outbreak season. A construction site where cut-proof gloves and a wash station mean fewer ER visits. A village where a handwashing station outside a birthing room becomes as routine as a blood pressure cuff. A world where antibiotics still work when we need them most because we used them less when we did not.

In the end, the story of antibiotics and humanity is not only about brilliant discoveries and daring rescues. It is also about ordinary people practicing ordinary care. We will always share this planet with microbes. We can meet them with fear, or we can meet them with habits that honor life.

Choose the habit. Choose the small act. Choose the simple thing done well, again and again.

Close the tap, dry your hands, and carry on. The next chapter of this story belongs to all of us, written in clean palms, tended wounds, and vaccination cards tucked into wallets and phone photos. If we keep choosing prevention, more children will grow up strong, more elders will watch sunsets from their porches, and the medicines that once felt like miracles will remain powerful enough to help the next patient who truly needs them. That is hope made practical. That is responsibility made light enough to share. And that is the power of simple habits.

Key ideas
- Prevention beats treatment—every time.
- Small daily habits and vaccines reduce the need for antibiotics.

Do this — Readers
- Stay current on vaccines.
- Wash hands, clean electronic devices, clean wounds promptly, use dental care, and manage chronic diseases.
- For procedures: Ask about infection-prevention steps you can take.

Do this — Clinicians

- Close vaccination gaps during sick visits; prescribe prevention (e.g., fluoride, wound care).
- Optimize peri-procedural prophylaxis—right drug, right dose, right timing, and stop after incision closure unless guidelines say otherwise.
- Empower patients with checklists and return-precaution scripts.
- Clean your stethoscopes between patients and let them know you did.

Conversation starters

- "Which vaccines am I due for?"
- "What can I do at home to prevent this from returning?"

Epilogue

Miracles and Consequences

On the kind of evening when the sky holds its breath, a nurse moves from room to room, rubbing sanitizer into her palms until it squeaks. Across town, a father rinses a scrape under the tap and hums twenty seconds of a song his kids know by heart. In a small apartment, someone opens a window to let the room breathe, then checks a vaccine card tucked behind a family photo. None of these moments feels like history, yet they are the story we have written together.

You have met so many people in these pages. Christine learning the edges of a new quiet. Ken blinking through a blur that might have taken more than sight. Miguel, whose world narrowed to silence, then widened again through community. Bob discovering that a routine surgery can become a battle and still be won. Amina in Khulna, her mother Sima, steadying a small hand and a brave new habit. Van bringing home a microbe he never saw, and a team learning, step by step, how to treat the next traveler better. Alina finding her way out of fear with a water bottle and a timer. Dr. Arun pausing at a sink because a promise matters. Gladys in Toronto, lacing garden boots and tending the fence that is her own skin. Chelsey in Florida, holding her daughter close, then holding a community together with a steady story.

Their lives did not change because of one grand gesture. They changed because of small decisions, stacked like bricks, that turned into shelter. Less when less is enough. More only when more is needed. Clean hands. Tended skin. Air that moves. Water that is safe. Vaccines that travel farther than viruses can. A medicine cabinet with fewer leftovers and more restraint. A clinic that pairs checklists with kindness. A hospital that treats a sink like a piece of lifesaving equipment. A neighborhood that sees prevention not as nagging, but as care.

Now the hard truth. Antibiotic resistance is not a distant rumble. It is here. Bacteria that were easy to treat a generation ago are harder to tame today. Millions of families have felt the cost. The burden is not shared evenly. A child in a low-income setting is far more likely to die from a resistant infection than a child with ready access to clean water, reliable power, and stocked pharmacies. That inequity should stop us in our tracks.

Yet this is not a chapter about despair. It is a chapter about the tools we already hold and the tools coming into our hands. We know that careful use of antibiotics slows resistance. We know that clean water, sanitation, ventilation, and vaccination prevent infections before they start. We know that simple habits in homes and hospitals change outcomes. And we are beginning to see how fast-moving science, including AI, can help us do all of this better.

In a growing number of hospitals, stewardship does not lean on memory alone. Electronic records nudge a clinician toward a narrower drug when the culture result lands. Bedside apps turn dense guidelines into simple choices. Algorithms flag a patient who is ready to stop antibiotics at day five, not day ten, and free a bed a day earlier. Rapid diagnostics, some driven by machine learning, identify the likely bug from a tiny sample in hours rather than days, so treatment fits the target instead of guessing wide. Public health teams use real-time dashboards to spot clusters early and move resources before an outbreak becomes a headline. Supply chains adjust when forecasting models predict vaccine demand in a coming season. None of this replaces judgment. It supports it, and it buys time.

These are reasons to be hopeful. Not because the threat is small, but because our response can be practical, humane, and smarter every month than it was the month before.

A Collective Responsibility

If there is one lesson to carry forward, it is that stewardship is not a specialist's ritual. It is a shared promise. Stewardship means using a precious drug in a way that leaves it useful for the next patient. It is empathy you can measure. It protects the person in the bed next door and the child who will need these medicines ten years from now.

Everyone has a role.

Patients and families can ask clear questions before asking for a prescription. *What is the most likely cause of this illness? If it is viral, what helps while my body heals? If an antibiotic is needed, what is the narrowest option, and how many days are truly enough?* Choosing not to take an antibiotic for a cold is not doing nothing. It is an act of care for yourself and for others. Keeping vaccines up to date, staying home when contagious, washing hands well, and tending small wounds early all reduce the infections that would have required antibiotics at all.

Clinicians carry a different weight. First, do no harm now includes future harm. Every prescription balances the needs of the person in front of you with the needs of the many you will never meet. Good stewardship looks like choosing the right drug at the right dose for the right number of days, then stopping on time. It looks like talking with the parent who came for a quick fix and leaving them with a plan that works without one. It looks like welcoming the nudge from the electronic record that says, this culture supports a narrower choice, or, your patient meets criteria to stop. AI can help here, not as a judge, but as a quiet second set of eyes.

Hospital leaders and policymakers set the stage. Fund stewardship teams and infection prevention staff. Make hand hygiene and device care easy to do every time. Support rapid diagnostics and the data systems that tie them to bedside choices. Regulate over-the-counter sales where misuse is common, and improve access where lifesaving drugs are out of reach. Invest in clean water, sanitation, and ventilation. Back vaccination campaigns that keep wards calm in the winter and classrooms open all year. Create incentives for new antibiotics and for alternatives that reduce the need for them. Use data to spot gaps and to direct help where it will matter most.

Think of these choices not as limits, but as gifts we pass along. Waiting a day to see if you improve without antibiotics. Picking the narrow drug. Stopping at five days when you are stable. These are small acts that, multiplied millions of times, extend the life of medicines we cannot replace quickly. The parallel with clean air and safe water is real. Antibiotic effectiveness is a shared resource. We inherited it. We can preserve it.

Innovation and Hope

On another night when the sky is quiet, a lab light clicks on. Someone in a white coat opens a laptop—not to scroll but to ask a model a question. *Which of these hundreds of compounds is worth a closer look?* The machine does not cure anyone. It suggests. It shortens the path. Across town, a nurse scans a barcode at a bedside, and a small alert appears: *Narrow your antibiotic now, the culture is back.* The nurse and physician read, think, choose, and a patient avoids a broad-spectrum drug they do not need. In a clinic on the edge of a crowded city, a mouth is swabbed, the swab goes into a hand-held box, and a tiny screen answers in hours, not days. This is a known bug and will respond to a simple antibiotic. The patient goes home sooner.

New tools are arriving. Bacteriophages (phages): The tiny viruses that infect and kill bacteria have been used in medicine since before antibiotics were invented, but now they are making a high-tech comeback. In labs, phages are being engineered and selected to act as living antibiotics, trained to hunt down specific bacteria that have become resistant to all other drugs. Unlike broad-spectrum antibiotics, which can wipe out beneficial bacteria along with the bad ones, phages work like laser-guided missiles, sparing the "good" microbes in our bodies while destroying the harmful ones. This precision could mean treating an infection without upsetting the body's microbiome or causing the collateral damage we see with antibiotics.

Phage therapy has already scored dramatic victories in individual cases where patients had no other hope, and clinical trials are underway to test its broader efficacy. It's a story that brings us full circle: using nature's own bacterium-killers, now bolstered by modern science, to cure where traditional antibiotics cannot.

The revolutionary gene-editing tool CRISPR, famous for its potential to rewrite DNA, is being repurposed to fight infection. Scientists are designing CRISPR-based antimicrobials that can zero in on bacteria's genetic code and disable the very genes that make them resistant or virulent.

Imagine a future where, instead of bombarding a bacterium with a drug, we send in a microscopic tool that chops up the resistance genes, effectively disarming the superbug from within. Early research has shown this can work in petri dishes; the challenge now is delivering such gene-editing therapies to the site of infection in a living patient. If achieved, it could open an era of "smart" antibiotics that leave good bacteria unscathed and target only the bad actors at the molecular level.

Other scientists are attacking the problem with nano-technology. They are crafting nano-scale materials, tiny particles far smaller than a cell, that can punch holes in bacterial membranes or deliver toxic payloads to bacterial cells without harming human tissue.

These nanoparticle-based therapies could be coated on surgical instruments or wound dressings to prevent infections, or injected to clear bacteria hiding in places traditional drugs struggle to reach. Meanwhile, biochemists are exploring anti-microbial peptides, which are essentially miniature proteins found in nature (for example, in our own immune system or in frog skin) that have the ability to destroy bacteria.

By tweaking these peptides or designing new ones, researchers hope to create medicines that bacteria won't shrug off easily. Some peptides poke lethal holes in bacterial walls, while others interfere with critical bacterial functions; importantly, they often work in ways entirely different from classical antibiotics, meaning they can bypass existing resistance mechanisms.

In diagnostics, teams are working hard and fast to develop diagnostic tools that move out of the central labs to carts, hands, and pockets, so we can make point-of-care diagnoses and decisions to treat the right infection at the right hour with the right drug.

Policy and design are part of this story, too. Smarter ventilation keeps indoor air from holding disease in place. Safer staffing ratios give caregivers enough minutes to wash, to teach, to check. Data dashboards show hot spots early so schools, shelters, and long-term care can respond before the curve rises. Supply chains borrow lessons from weather forecasting to get vaccines and antibiotics where they will be needed, not where they were needed last year.

Education is changing. Residents carry quieter confidence because the guideline is in their pocket, and the culture supports saying, I am stopping at five days. Parents hear a clear plan for a viral illness and leave with tools, not pills. Farmers use vaccines and hygiene to keep herds healthy, and their buyers reward them for it. Communities learn that clean water and sanitation are not charity, but infrastructure that pays for itself in calmer hospitals and stronger economies.

None of these advances replaces the simple habits that carried us through this book. They amplify them. A rapid test makes it easier to withhold an antibiotic when it will not help. A stewardship alert gives cover to a busy doctor who wants to stop on time. A vaccine forecast softens the peak that would have filled a ward. Innovation and restraint pull in the same direction. One buys time for the other.

Stewardship belongs here, not as a lecture, but as the way we love each other with medicine. We use enough, we stop on time, we save the strongest drugs for the moments that truly call for them. Think of antibiotics like a river that runs through a town. When it's protected, it runs clear and sustains everyone downstream. When it's overused or polluted, it turns murky—and the harm spreads far beyond the original source. In this era, stewardship is not only a duty. It is a chance to be kind in a measurable way.

The horizon is not empty. We will see more rapid tests that guide treatment at the first visit. We will see decision tools that lower the noise and lift the signal at the point of care. We will see materials and coatings that make devices less welcoming to germs. We will see phages and new molecules clear infections that defeated yesterday's best drugs. We will see school lessons that make hygiene and vaccine literacy as ordinary as multiplication tables. We will see stronger global agreements that keep lifesaving antibiotics out of over-the-counter bins and in the hands of trained prescribers, while making sure the right drugs reach places that don't have them.

There will be setbacks. There always are. Bacteria evolve. Funding ebbs and flows. New tools will need careful trials and careful rules. But we are no longer walking in the dark. We have maps. We have stories. We have proof that less can be enough, and that prevention is a gift that keeps on giving. So here is how this book ends, and how your part begins.

Wash your hands with intention. Tend small wounds early. Keep air moving where you live and work. Stay current on vaccines and ask questions until you feel steady. Use antibiotics only when they are truly needed, and stop when the job is done. If you care for patients, make these choices visible so others can follow you. If you lead teams, build systems that make the right thing easy on a hard day. If you shape policy, fund the quiet things that save the most lives, clean water, sanitation, ventilation, vaccination, and the stewardship teams who keep our medicines strong.

You will not see the infections you prevent. You will see something else. A child at school on a Tuesday who would have been in bed. A grandparent at a birthday instead of a ward. A nurse who leaves on time because the unit is calmer. A pharmacy shelf where the strongest drugs still work for the person who truly needs them.

Close the tap. Dry your hands. Keep the habits. Welcome the new tools. Use them with care. Pass them on stronger than you found them.

That is how hope becomes practice. That is how practice becomes culture. And that is how, together, we keep writing a future where more people heal, fewer people suffer, and the fragile miracle of antibiotics endures.

Use antibiotics like a shared inheritance: only when needed, and always with care.

Small Harms, Big Consequences

People hear "side effects" and imagine lightning strikes: the rare reaction, the headline complication, the thing that makes doctors lower their voices.

But most antibiotic harm is quieter than that.

It shows up as a mouth that burns, a body that can't tolerate sunlight, a throat that feels scraped raw, a child's smile that looks different in photos, a strange blue-gray stain that wasn't there before. These aren't usually life-threatening. That is exactly why they get dismissed. And that dismissal has consequences.

Because these are the harms that make patients do very human things. They:

- stop early
- skip doses
- take the next pill different than prescribed
- borrow leftovers
- decide they can't tolerate antibiotics and avoid care next time
- lose trust in the person who prescribed the antibiotic

This chapter is not meant to scare anyone away from antibiotics. It's meant to keep people on the right medicine, in the right way, for the right length of time, with fewer avoidable detours. Consider it a field guide. Not to fear. To foresight.

Each section follows the same path: What it feels like. Why it happens. What to do. How to prevent it next time.

1. Yeast overgrowth: thrush + vulvovaginal candidiasis

What it feels like

Sometimes the infection improves and the body still feels worse.

In the mouth: soreness, a cottony taste, cracking at the corners of the lips, and creamy white patches on the tongue or cheeks that wipe off and leave raw skin beneath.

In the vagina: itching, burning, irritation, and a thick discharge that can make a person feel dirty even when they are doing everything "right. "

These aren't dramatic symptoms. They're just relentless. And they are one of the most common reasons people quietly decide, *I'm not taking another pill.*

Why it happens

Yeast lives with us. It's not a moral failure. It's biology.

Antibiotics, especially broader-spectrum ones, thin out the helpful bacteria that keep yeast contained. Once that balance is disturbed, Candida takes advantage of the open space. The antibiotic doesn't create yeast out of nowhere. It removes the neighbors that keep yeast from moving in.

What to do

Call when symptoms begin during or soon after an antibiotic course. Don't wait for discomfort to ripen into misery and panic.

If you're immunocompromised, pregnant, diabetic, or prone to recurrent yeast infections, call early. The threshold should be lower.

If you can't swallow, can't keep fluids down, or you have fever with mouth sores, get evaluated promptly.

How to prevent it next time

Before starting antibiotics, ask: "Should I watch for thrush or yeast symptoms with this medication? "

If you've had yeast issues before, say it upfront. That history matters.

Don't self-treat in the dark with random leftovers. A simple, timely plan prevents a spiral.

2. Photosensitivity: Doxycycline and TMP-SMX

What it feels like

A sunburn that doesn't match the day.

You step outside the way you always do. A walk to the mailbox. A quick errand. A drive with the window cracked. And by evening your skin feels hot, tight, and angry. Sometimes it blisters. Sometimes it looks like a rash and you wonder if you're allergic.

This harm is "small" until it cancels a vacation, interrupts work, or makes someone stop the medication in frustration.

Why it happens

Certain antibiotics change how skin responds to ultraviolet light. The rules of sunlight are rewritten while the medicine is in your system. It's not vanity. It's chemistry.

What to do

If you develop an intense sunburn-like reaction while taking one of these antibiotics, assume the medication is part of the story and call for guidance.

If you have blistering, facial swelling, fever, or a rapidly spreading rash, get evaluated. Not every skin reaction is benign. Don't "test it" again the next day. That experiment rarely ends well.

How to prevent it next time

Minimize sun exposure during the course. Use protective clothing and sunscreen. Avoid tanning beds entirely.

Plan ahead. If someone is starting these antibiotics before a beach week, outdoor job, sports tournament, or long road trip, that timing should be part of the prescription conversation.

3. Pill esophagitis: the preventable throat injury

What it feels like

It can feel like sudden heartburn with teeth. Or like swallowing glass.

People describe sharp chest pain, pain with swallowing, and the sense that something is stuck. It often begins after taking a pill right before bed, or dry-swallowing with a sip of water that isn't enough.

Most people who get this weren't reckless. They were tired.

Why it happens

Some pills don't slide cleanly into the stomach. They linger in the esophagus. They dissolve there. They irritate the lining like a chemical burn. If you lie down immediately, gravity stops helping.

What to do

If you have severe chest pain, trouble swallowing, vomiting, or an inability to keep fluids down, get evaluated.

If symptoms are mild but persistent, call. The fix may be simple, but the injury is real. Don't keep forcing doses through pain without guidance.

How to prevent it next time

This is one of the most preventable antibiotic harms in the entire book:

- Take the pill with a full glass of water.
- Stay upright for at least thirty minutes after swallowing.
- Avoid taking it right before sleep.

4. Tooth staining and discoloration: the visible harm that changes behavior

This is where we have to be honest and careful. There is classic, well-established permanent-tooth discoloration associated with tetracycline use during tooth development. That's real, and it belongs in the conversation before the first dose.

There are also reports of tooth discoloration with other antibiotics, including amoxicillin–clavulanate (Augmentin), but that evidence is more variable. When it happens, it may be surface staining rather than true developmental staining. The experience still matters because it's visible.

What it feels like

A parent notices it in the bathroom mirror. A new yellow-brown tint. A change in the way teeth are photographed. It's not dangerous in the moment. But it can feel like a betrayal: We treated an infection and got a new problem we can see.

Why it happens

There are different mechanisms:

- Tetracyclines administered during tooth development can integrate into developing enamel and dentin, resulting in permanent color changes.
- Other antibiotics may be associated with discoloration through surface staining, changes in oral flora, or indirect effects. The evidence varies by drug.

What to do

Tell your prescriber and your dentist. This is a shared lane
If it's a child, ask: "Is there a narrower option for next time? "
Don't let shame or blame drive the conversation. This is about
planning, not fault.

How to prevent it next time

For young children and pregnant patients, tetracyclines require extra caution because the risk is known and
preventable.

For drugs like Augmentin, you don't need fear, but you can
set expectations. Rare things happen. If you notice changes,
tell us early.

5. Minocycline hyperpigmentation: when treatment leaves a mark

What it feels like

A bruise that doesn't behave like a bruise.

Blue-gray or brown patches appear on the skin. Sometimes
the gums darken. Scars look different. Nails can shift color. It
can be subtle at first, then suddenly obvious once you know
what you're seeing. The fear isn't only cosmetic. The fear is
permanence.

Why it happens

With prolonged exposure, minocycline can deposit pig-
ment in tissues. Some patterns correlate with cumulative dose
and long-term therapy.

What to do

If discoloration occurs during minocycline therapy, report
it promptly.
Ask: "Is this still the best option, or can we switch? "

If discoloration is accompanied by systemic symptoms such as fatigue, dark urine, or jaundice, seek evaluation. Don't assume every visible change is purely "skin deep. "

How to prevent it next time

Long-term antibiotics should never be "set it and forget it. "If a drug is known to leave visible, sometimes lasting changes, that belongs in the consent conversation, not the footnotes.

6. Intracranial hypertension is rare, but don't miss it

What it feels like

A headache that has a personality. Not the typical headache of dehydration or stress. The kind that presses behind the eyes. The kind that presents with blurred vision, double vision, or a pulsating sensation in the eyes. Sometimes there is ringing in the ears. Sometimes nausea joins the party.

Why it happens

We don't always know exactly why. We do know it's a recognized adverse effect of tetracyclines, and it can persist even after stopping the drug.

What to do

Stop taking tetracycline and call the office promptly if you develop a severe headache with visual symptoms.

If you have vision loss, a severe, persistent headache, or neurologic symptoms, seek medical attention. If you're taking isotretinoin, that combination matters. Don't let it be missed.

How to prevent it next time

You don't prevent rare events by living in fear. You prevent them by clearly identifying warning signs once, so the patient can recognize the pattern early.

A prescription should come with one sentence that sticks: "If you get a bad headache with blurred vision on this medicine, don't push through it. Call. "

7. Blood count suppression on prolonged therapy: Why monitoring matters

What it feels like

This one can be sneaky.

It can feel like fatigue that doesn't make sense. Easy bruising. Mouth sores. A sore throat that lingers. New fevers. Sometimes, nothing at all until a lab quietly waves a flag.

Why it happens

Some antibiotics can suppress bone marrow function or trigger immune-mediated decreases in blood cells, especially when therapy extends into weeks. The risk is not only the molecule. The risk is time on the molecule, particularly outside the hospital, where missed labs are easy, and symptoms get blamed on "recovery. "

What to do

If you're on prolonged therapy and develop fever, sore throat, mouth ulcers, unusual bruising, bleeding gums, or profound fatigue, call your doctor promptly.

If you missed scheduled labs, don't shrug. Reschedule quickly.

Ask for clarity: "Who is monitoring the labs, and how will I be told about results? "

How to prevent it next time

Prolonged therapy should come with a written monitoring plan, not a vague reassurance. Patients should know what's being checked, how often, and who owns follow-up. Clinicians should treat missed labs as a safety issue, not a nuisance.

Final checklist: when to call, when to go

This is the simplest safety net I know: a short list that reduces regret. It doesn't replace clinical judgment. It prevents delay.

> **Go now (urgent care or the nearest emergency department) if you have:**
> - Trouble breathing, swelling of lips/tongue/ throat, or widespread hives
> - A rash with blistering, peeling skin, or fever
> - Severe watery or bloody diarrhea, especially with fever or abdominal pain
> - Severe headache with blurred vision, double vision, or vision loss while on a tetracycline
> - Inability to swallow fluids, persistent vomiting, or signs of dehydration

Most people don't stop taking antibiotics because of a headline complication. They stop because the medicine makes daily life unpleasant in small, relentless ways.

Nausea that steals appetite. Loose stools that make you afraid to leave the house. A metallic taste that turns every meal into cardboard. A mouth that feels coated. A yeast infection that arrives just as the original problem starts to improve.

These are not the dramatic harms that fill warning labels, but they are the harms that shape behavior. They decide whether a teenager finishes the course, whether a parent gives the next dose, whether a patient trusts the next prescription, and whether someone saves leftovers "just in case. "

If this chapter has one message, it is this: Don't suffer in silence and don't quit in secret. Call. Ask for a plan. Sometimes the answer is simple: take it with food, change the timing, treat the yeast early, switch to a narrower option, shorten the course when it's safe, or step down from IV to pills sooner than expected.

Strong medicine can be a gift. But even gifts deserve clear instructions.

And when we name the small harms honestly, we spare patients the lonely kind of regret.

If you made it this far, you already understand the point. Antibiotics are not villains. They are some of the most powerful gifts medicine has ever held.

But power deserves humility. A good plan isn't only the right drug. It's the right dose, the right duration, the right route, and the right conversation.

When we name the small harms, we don't weaken the case for antibiotics. We strengthen it. We help everyone finish what matters, avoid what doesn't, and keep trust intact for the moment when the stakes are higher.

May we use these medicines with wisdom. May we listen closely to the people carrying the cost. And may healing, when it comes, arrive with as little collateral damage as possible.

Appendix

Antibiotics—The Questions That Prevent Harm

Antibiotics save lives. They also carry costs that most people never hear about until the cost shows up in their own body.

This appendix is not meant to turn you into a doctor. It is meant to give you language. The right questions do two things at once: They protect you from avoidable harm, and they help your clinician make the safest plan with you.

Use these questions the way you would use a seatbelt. Not because you expect a crash, but because you respect what can happen when things move fast.

Urgent care / outpatient

These are the moments when antibiotics are most often started quickly, sometimes before the full picture is clear.

"What infection are we treating, and how sure are we?" Ask what the diagnosis is, what makes them confident, and what else it could be.

"Is an antibiotic necessary today, or is watchful waiting safe?" For many common problems, time, fluids, pain control, and a follow-up plan are safer than a reflex prescription.

"If we do treat, what is the narrowest option for this likely bug?" This pushes the plan away from "strongest" and toward "most appropriate. "

"What are the top side effects you're most worried about for me?" Not a long list. The two or three that fit your age, kidneys, heart rhythm, other medications, pregnancy status, allergies, or past reactions.

Hospital admission

In the hospital, antibiotics are often started before cultures return. This is appropriate, but it should never remain a guessing game.

"What cultures or tests are we using to confirm the infection?" Blood cultures, urine culture, imaging, viral testing. If there is no plan to confirm, the antibiotic plan is often less stable.

"What is the plan to narrow or stop antibiotics when results come back?" Ask for a timeline: "When will we reassess? Tomorrow? In forty-eight hours?" De-escalation should be a scheduled event, not a vague intention.

"How long do you expect I'll need antibiotics, and what would make it shorter or longer?" Duration matters. Ask for the expected range and the factors that change it (source control, response, organism, immune status).

"Are any of my other medications or conditions a problem with this antibiotic?" This is where you catch real-world harms: warfarin interactions, QT prolongation, kidney dosing, seizure risk, allergy history, and high-risk combinations.

Discharge on prolonged therapy

This is where harm often sneaks in: not because the antibiotic is wrong, but because the plan is fragile once you leave the building.

"What is our goal and stop rule?" Ask for one clear sentence: "We're treating X until Y happens, then we stop." The goal may be symptom resolution, lab normalization, imaging improvement, or a fixed duration backed by evidence.

"How will we monitor for harm, and who owns the results?" Get specifics: Which labs, how often, where they are drawn, who reviews them, and how you'll be contacted. If no one "owns" the results, problems get missed.

"Can any of this be done by mouth instead of IV? And if not now, then when?" If you are going home on IV antibiotics, ask what milestones allow oral step-down. IV is sometimes necessary, but it should rarely be the default forever.

"What symptoms should make me call today, and what symptoms mean I should seek care right away?" Ask for a short red-flag list tailored to your plan. If you are on OPAT, make sure it includes line-related warnings (fever/chills, new arm swelling/pain, redness/drainage, line malfunction).

A final note

If you ask these questions and your clinician welcomes them, that is a good sign. If they look rushed, ask anyway. The goal is not to challenge expertise. The goal is to make the plan safer. Because the best antibiotic decision is not only about killing bacteria. It is also about keeping the patient whole while you do it.

Acknowledgments

This book carries my name on the cover, but it was never a solo effort. Beyond the Cure was shaped by people who read early drafts when the story was still rough, challenged my assumptions, sharpened my language, and reminded me why this message matters. I am deeply grateful to everyone who helped bring these pages to life. The names below are shared in no particular order.

I want to begin with Emeritus Professor Joseph Garner, MD, my first editor, who read the raw draft and loved it. He stepped into the earliest version with generosity and seriousness, and his thoughtful comments helped me see the book more clearly from the start.

Some support changes the weight of the work. Ronald Nahass, MD, MHCM, FIDSA, President of the Infectious Diseases Society of America and interim CEO/President of ID Care, trusted this message and offered a generous endorsement when it mattered most. Brad Spellberg, MD, wrote the foreword without a second thought, lending clarity, credibility, and conviction to the story I was trying to tell.

I am thankful to Rosanna Li, PharmD, an infectious diseases–trained pharmacist, who edited several chapters with a careful eye and the practical wisdom that only daily stewardship work can give. Your feedback strengthened both the science and the sense.

To Drs. Kevin Dieckhaus, Lisa Chirch, and David Banach, thank you for reviewing the manuscript and for endorsing the book. Your support affirmed the value of this project, and your perspective helped me keep the clinical voice grounded while still speaking to everyday readers. Kevin, your global perspective broadened the book's frame and reminded me that the consequences of antibiotics do not stop at any border.

To Dr. Mohammed Shams, thank you for your invaluable support while I put this together. You provided the environment and the time to write, which is no small gift in modern medicine.

To Dr. Ajay Kumar, your support is greatly appreciated. Some people are gifted with the skill to lead, and you are one of them. You saw the potential in this book and responded quickly, even on weekends.

To Mrs. Gina Coleman and Dr. Yaw Perbi, for the support and endorsement. Your voice will take this book places and transform many lives.

To my colleagues in infectious diseases, thank you for reading sections, offering encouragement, and pushing this work forward: Drs. Stephanie Wright, Sarah Banks, Zoheir Khan, Jesse Serrins, Carol Halasan, and Brenton Nash. In a field where the work is heavy and the days are full, your willingness to pause and engage with the manuscript meant a great deal. And to the seasoned academic hospitalist, Dr. Madura Saravanan, your ideas are just brilliant.

To Dr. Ulysses Wu, thank you for your support. And to Paul Anthony, MD, my colleague and friend, thank you for the encouragement and edits. Your steady belief in this project helped me keep going when the finish line felt far.

I am grateful to Michael McConnell, my copyeditor, for making my work more translatable to general readers. You helped preserve the voice while improving clarity, pacing, and precision. That balance is tricky to pull off, and you did it with skill and care.

To Dr. Yaw Ampadu and Mr. Obeng Gyebi, thank you for transforming the book cover and enhancing its shelf appeal.

You gave the story a visual identity that invites readers in before they've read a single line.

To Mr. Emmanuel Sakyi, thank you for transforming this book into a website (beyondthecurebook.com) for a global audience.

Some support is quieter but just as essential. To Ms. Kenya Humphrey, my administrative assistant and resident "detective," thank you for the behind-the-scenes help that kept a hundred small tasks from becoming obstacles. Your reliability made progress possible.

To Dr. Ophelia Chapman and Mrs. Sheela Awuah Fosu, thank you for your invaluable support throughout this process. I felt your care, your steadiness, and your encouragement more times than I can count.

To my parents and siblings, thank you for the support, prayers, and constant reminders of where I come from. A book like this is built on a lifetime of investment from family long before the first chapter is written.

To my children, thank you for sacrificing some "Daddy time" so this book could move forward. I know what it costs when a parent is present, but also thinking about a paragraph, a deadline, or a final revision. I see that sacrifice, and I do not take it lightly.

And to my wife, thank you for reading the multiple drafts, for suggesting comments, and for being an honest sounding board from the beginning. She helped me write for the real world, not just the medical world.

To everyone who offered feedback, prayed, checked in, covered a clinical need, or simply kept cheering when the work felt endless, thank you. I hope this book honors your support by helping readers make wiser choices, ask better questions, and protect what antibiotics were meant to preserve.

Bibliography

Chapter 1. Poor Liver

- National Institute of Diabetes and Digestive and Kidney Diseases. Liver Disease. Bethesda, MD: NIDDK, n.d. Accessed November 1, 2025.
  https://www.niddk.nih.gov/health-information/liver-disease

- National Institute of Diabetes and Digestive and Kidney Diseases. LiverTox: Clinical and Research Information on Drug-Induced Liver Injury. Bethesda, MD: NIDDK/National Library of Medicine, 2012–. Accessed November 1, 2025.
  https://www.ncbi.nlm.nih.gov/books/NBK548241/

- National Institute of Diabetes and Digestive and Kidney Diseases. "Amoxicillin–Clavulanate." In LiverTox. Bethesda, MD: NIDDK/National Library of Medicine, 2012–. Accessed November 1, 2025.
  https://www.ncbi.nlm.nih.gov/books/NBK548517/

- Chalasani, Naga, et al. "Causes, Clinical Features, and Outcomes from a Prospective Study of Drug-Induced Liver Injury in the United States." Gastroenterology 135, no. 6 (2008): 1924–34.
  https://doi.org/10.1053/j.gastro.2008.09.011

- Fontana, Robert J. "Pathogenesis of Idiosyncratic Drug-Induced Liver Injury and Clinical Perspectives." Gastroenterology 146, no. 4 (2014): 914–28.
  https://doi.org/10.1053/j.gastro.2013.12.043

- Stine, Jonathan G., and Naga Chalasani. "Chronic Liver Injury Induced by Drugs: A Systematic Review." Liver International 35, no. 11 (2015): 2343–49.
  https://doi.org/10.1111/liv.12968

- Andrade, Raúl J., and Paul M. Tulkens. "Hepatic Safety of Antibiotics Used in Primary Care." Journal of Antimicrobial Chemotherapy 66, no. 7 (2011): 1431–46.
  https://doi.org/10.1093/jac/dkr159

- Björnsson, Einar S. "Drug-Induced Liver Injury Due to Antibiotics." Scandinavian Journal of Gastroenterology 44, no. 4 (2009): 447–58.
  https://doi.org/10.1080/003C5520802C00S3S

- Torgersen, Jessie, Alyssa K. Mezochow, Craig W. Newcomb, et al. "Severe Acute Liver Injury After Hepatotoxic Medication Initiation in Real-World Data." JAMA Internal Medicine 184, no. 8 (2024): 943–52.
  https://jamanetwork.com/journalsjamainternalmedicine/
  fullarticle/2820267

- U.S. Food and Drug Administration. AUGMENTIN® (amoxicillin and clavulanate potassium) Tablets, for Oral Use—Prescribing Information. Initial U.S. Approval 1984; revised December 2024. Accessed November 1, 2025.
  https://www.accessdata.fda.gov/drugsatfda_docs/
  label/2024/050564s055,050575 s051,050597s042lbl.pdf.

- Science Museum Group (London). "Amoxicillin Discovered, United Kingdom, 1972." Science Museum Group Collection. Accessed November 1, 2025.
  https://collection.sciencemuseumgroup.org.uk/objects/co68163
  Reading, C., and M. Cole. "Clavulanic Acid: A Beta-Lactamase-
  Inhibiting Beta-Lactam from Streptomyces clavuligerus."
  Antimicrobial Agents and Chemotherapy 11, no. 5 (1977): 852–57.

- World Health Organization. Latent Tuberculosis Infection: Updated and Consolidated Guidelines for Programmatic Management. Geneva: WHO, 2018. Accessed November 1, 2025.
  https://iris.who.int/bitstream/handle/10CC5/2C0233/ S78S24155023S-eng.pdf

- Centers for Disease Control and Prevention. Latent Tuberculosis Infection: A Guide for Primary Healthcare Providers. Atlanta: CDC, 2020 (web edition). Accessed November 1, 2025.
  https://www.cdc.gov/tb/publications/ltbi/guide.htm

- Saukkonen, J. J., D. L. Cohn, R. M. Jasmer, et al. "An Official ATS Statement: Hepatotoxicity of Antituberculosis Therapy." American Journal of Respiratory and Critical Care Medicine 174, no. 8 (2006): 935–52.
  https://doi.org/10.11C4/rccm.200510-1CCCST

- Nolan, C. M., S. V. Goldberg, and S. E. Buskin. "Hepatotoxicity Associated with Isoniazid Preventive Therapy: A 7-Year Survey from a Public Health Tuberculosis Clinic." JAMA 281, no. 11 (1999): 1014–18.
  https://doi.org/10.1001/jama.281.11.1014

- Steele, M. A., R. F. Burk, and R. M. Des Prez. "Toxic Hepatitis with Isoniazid and Rifampin: A Meta-Analysis." Chest 99, no. 2 (1991): 465–71.
  https://doi.org/10.1378/chest. SS.2.4C5

- Pande, J. N., S. P. Singh, G. C. Khilnani, et al. "Risk Factors for Hepatotoxicity from Antituberculosis Drugs: A Case-Control Study." Thorax 51, no. 2 (1996): 132–36.
  https://doi.org/10.113C/thx.51.2.132

- Russo, Michael W., John A. Galanko, Rohit Shrestha, Michael W. Fried, and Paul B. Watkins. "Liver Transplantation for Acute Liver Failure from Drug-Induced Liver Injury in the United States." Liver Transplantation 10, no. 8 (2004): 1018–23.
  https://doi.org/10.1002/lt.20200

- Watkins, Paul B. "Idiosyncratic Liver Injury: Challenges and Approaches." Toxicologic Pathology 33, no. 1 (2005): 1–5.
  https://doi.org/10.1080/01S2C2305S08S01S5

- U.S. Food and Drug Administration. New Drug Application 20-7C0: Alatrofloxacin/Trovafloxacin—Medical Review Excerpts on Hepatic Safety. Silver Spring, MD: FDA, 1997–1999. Accessed November 1, 2025.
  https://www.accessdata.fda.gov/drugsatfda_docs/nda/S7/0207C0a_medr_P27.pdf

- MedlinePlus. "Amoxicillin and Clavulanate." U.S. National Library of Medicine. Accessed November 1, 2025.
  https://medlineplus.gov/druginfo/meds/aC85024.html

Chapter 2. Gut Feeling

- Fischer, M., B. Sipe, Y.-W. Cheng, et al. "Fecal Microbiota Transplant in Severe and Severe-Complicated Clostridium difficile: A Promising Treatment Approach." Gut Microbes 8, no. 3 (2017): 289–302.
  https://doi.org/10.1080/19490976.2016.1273998

- Hall, I. C., and E. O'Toole. "Intestinal Flora in New-Born Infants: With a Description of a New Pathogenic Anaerobe, Bacillus difficilis." American Journal of Diseases of Children 49, no. 2 (1935): 390–402.
  https://doi.org/10.1001/archpedi.1935.01970020105010

- McDonald, L. C., D. N. Gerding, S. Johnson, et al. "Clinical Practice Guidelines for Clostridium difficile Infection in Adults and Children: 2017 Update by the Infectious Diseases Society of America (IDSA) and Society for Healthcare Epidemiology of America (SHEA)." Clinical Infectious Diseases 66, no. 7 (2018): e1–e48.
  https://doi.org/10.1093/cid/cix1085

- Hall, I. C., and E. O'Toole. "Further Studies on Bacillus difficilis." Journal of Infectious Diseases 60, no. 2 (1937): 223–31.
  https://doi.org/10.1093/infdis/60.2.223

- Skerman, V. B. D., V. McGowan, and P. H. A. Sneath, eds. Approved Lists of Bacterial Names (Amended). Washington, DC: ASM Press, 1989.
  https://www.ncbi.nlm.nih.gov/books/NBK814/

- Snyder, M. L. "The Normal Fecal Flora of Infants between Two Weeks and One Year of Age: Serial Studies." Journal of Infectious Diseases 66, no. 1 (1940): 1–16.
  https://doi.org/10.1093/infdis/66.1.1

- Smith, L. D. S., and E. O. King. "Occurrence of Clostridium difficile in Infections of Man." Journal of Bacteriology 84, no. 1 (1962): 65–67.
  https://doi.org/10.1128/JB.84.1.65-67.1962

- Sutter, V. L., and S. M. Finegold. "The Effect of Antimicrobial Agents on Human Fecal Flora: Studies with Cephalexin, Cyclacillin, and Clindamycin." Society for Applied Bacteriology Symposium Series 3, no. 0 (1974): 229–40.

- Freedberg, Daniel E., Ian D. P. Furuya, Bevin Cohen, Julian A. Abrams, and Elaine L. Larson. "Prior Antimicrobial Exposure of Hospital Room Occupants and Risk for Clostridium difficile Infection Among Subsequent Room Occupants." JAMA Internal Medicine 176, no. 11 (2016): 1801–1808. *https://jamanetwork.com/journals/jamainternalmedicine/article-abstract/2540123*

- Shaughnessy, Mary K., Erika Micielli, Amelia L. DePestel, et al. "Evaluation of Hospital Room Assignment and Acquisition of Clostridium difficile Infection." Infection Control & Hospital Epidemiology 32, no. 3 (2011): 201–206. *https://doi.org/10.108C/C58CCS*

- Witt, Lucy S., Jessica Howard-Anderson, Jennifer S. Jacob, Jesse T. Jacob, and Scott A. Fridkin. "Impact of Exposure to Hospital Beds Contaminated with Clostridioides difficile Spores on Risk of Hospital-Onset C. difficile Infection." Infection Control & Hospital Epidemiology (2024). *https://doi.org/10.1017/ice.2024.68*

- A. Fridkin. "Impact of Exposure to Hospital Beds Contaminated with Clostridioides difficile Spores on Risk of Hospital-Onset C. difficile Infection." Infection Control & Hospital Epidemiology (2024). *https://doi.org/10.1017/ice.2024.68*

- Rifkin, G. D., F. R. Fekety, J. Silva, and R. B. Sack. "Antibiotic-Induced Colitis: Implication of a Toxin Neutralized by Clostridium sordellii Antitoxin." The Lancet 310, no. 8048 (1977): 1103–6. *https://doi.org/10.1016/S0140-6736(77)90547-5*

- George, R. H., J. M. Symonds, F. Dimock, et al. "Identification of Clostridium difficile as a Cause of Pseudomembranous Colitis." British Medical Journal 1, no. 6114 (1978): 695.
https://doi.org/10.1136/bmj.1.6114.695

- Lance, G. W., Ellie J. C. Goldstein, Vera L. Sutter, Shelly L. Ludwig, and Sydney M. Finegold. "Ætiology of Antimicrobial-Agent-Associated Colitis." The Lancet 311, no. 8068 (1978): 802–3.
https://doi.org/10.1016/S0140-6736(78)93001-5

- Rodriguez, C., J. Van Broeck, B. Taminiau, M. Delmée, and G. Daube. "Clostridium difficile Infection: Early History, Diagnosis, and Molecular Strain Typing Methods." Microbial Pathogenesis 97 (2016): 59–78.
https://doi.org/10.1016/j.micpath.2016.05.018

- Farooq, P. D., N. H. Urrunaga, D. M. Tang, and E. C. von Rosenvinge. "Pseudomembranous Colitis." Disease-a-Month 61, no. 5 (2015): 181–206.
https://doi.org/10.1016/j.disamonth.2015.01.006

- Pépin, J., L. Valiquette, M.-E. Alary, et al. "Clostridium difficile-Associated Diarrhea in a Region of Quebec from 1991 to 2003: A Changing Pattern of Disease Severity." Canadian Medical Association Journal 171, no. 5 (2004): 466–72.
https://doi.org/10.1503/cmaj.1041104

- McDonald, L. C., M. Owings, and D. B. Jernigan. "Clostridium difficile Infection in Patients Discharged from US Short-Stay Hospitals, 1996-2003." Emerging Infectious Diseases 12, no. 3 (2006): 409–15.
https://doi.org/10.3201/eid1205.051064

- Reveles, K. R., G. C. Lee, N. K. Boyd, and C. R. Frei. "The Rise in Clostridium difficile Infection Incidence Among Hospitalized Adults in the United States: 2001-2010." American Journal of Infection Control 42, no. 10 (2014): 1028–32.
https://doi.org/10.1016/j.ajic.2014.06.011

- Lessa, F. C., Y. Mu, W. M. Bamberg, et al. "Burden of Clostridium difficile Infection in the United States." New England Journal of Medicine 372, no. 9 (2015): 825–34. *https://doi.org/10.1056/NEJMoa1408913*

- Centers for Disease Control and Prevention (CDC). Antibiotic Resistance Threats in the United States, 201S. Atlanta, GA: CDC, 2019.

Chapter 3: Allergic to the Cure

- American Academy of Allergy, Asthma C Immunology. "Drug Allergy." Accessed January 2, 2025.
  https://www.aaaai.org/conditions-treatments/allergies/drug-allergy

- American Academy of Pediatrics. "Antibiotic Stewardship." Last modified October 5, 2020.
  https://www.aap.org/en/patient-care/antibiotic-stewardship/

- Zagursky, Robert J., and Amanda M. Pisoni. "Penicillin Allergy: A Practical Guide for Clinicians." Cleveland Clinic Journal of Medicine 87, no. 5 (2020): 295–300.
  https://doi.org/10.3S4S/ccjm.87a.1811S

- Andrade, Raúl J., and Paul M. Tulkens. "Hepatic Safety of Antibiotics Used in Primary Care." Journal of Antimicrobial Chemotherapy 66, no. 7 (2011): 1431–46.
  https://doi.org/10.10S3/jac/dkr15S

- Aronson, Jeffrey K., ed. Side Effects of Drugs Annual: A Worldwide Yearly Survey of New Data in Adverse Drug Reactions. 38th ed. Amsterdam: Elsevier, 2016. Centers for Disease Control and Prevention. Antibiotic Resistance Threats in the United States, 2019. Atlanta: U.S. Department of Health and Human Services, CDC, 2019.
  https://www.cdc.gov/drugresistance/pdf/threats-report/2019-ar-threats-report-508.pdf

- Centers for Disease Control and Prevention. Antibiotic Resistance Threats in the United States, 201S. Atlanta: U.S. Department of Health and Human Services, CDC, 2019.
  https://www.cdc.gov/drugresistance/pdf/threats-report/201S-ar-threats-report-508.pdf

- Centers for Disease Control and Prevention. "Medication Safety Program: Facts and Statistics." Last modified March 1, 2022.
  https://www.cdc.gov/medication-safety/data-research/facts-stats/index.html

- Demoly, Pascal, and Jean-Christoph Pichler. "Drug Hypersensitivity Reactions: Classification and Management." *Allergy* 68, no. 7 (2013): 820–31.
  https://doi.org/10.1111/all.1212C

- Joint Task Force on Practice Parameters; American Academy of Allergy, Asthma C Immunology; American College of Allergy, Asthma C Immunology; Joint Council of Allergy, Asthma C Immunology. "Drug Allergy: An Updated Practice Parameter." *Annals of Allergy, Asthma & Immunology* 105, no. 4 (2010): 259–73.
  https://doi.org/10.101C/j.anai.2010.08.002

- Khan, David A., Aleena Banerji, Kimberly G. Blumenthal, Elizabeth J. Phillips, Roland Solensky, and colleagues. "Drug Allergy: A 2022 Practice Parameter Update." *Journal of Allergy and Clinical Immunology* 150, no. 6 (2022): 1333–93.
  https://doi.org/10.1016/j.jaci.2022.07.016

- Macy, Eric, and Caileigh Ngor. "Safely Diagnosing Clinically Significant Penicillin Allergy Using Penicillin Skin Testing and Oral Amoxicillin Challenge Testing." *JACI: In Practice* 1, no. 3 (2013): 258–63.
  https://doi.org/10.101C/j.jaip.2013.02.002

- Macy, Eric, and Thanai Pongdee. "Management of Patients with a History of Penicillin Allergy." *JACI: In Practice* 2, no. 3 (2014): 258–63.
  https://doi.org/10.101C/j.jaip.2014.02.005

- MedlinePlus. "Penicillin Allergy." U.S. National Library of Medicine. Accessed January 2, 2025.
  https://medlineplus.gov/ency/article/00081S.htm

- Naranjo, Carlos A., Usoa Busto, Edward M. Sellers, Philip Sandor, Ian Ruiz, Elizabeth A. Roberts, et al. "A Method for Estimating the Probability of Adverse Drug Reactions." *Clinical Pharmacology & Therapeutics* 30, no. 2 (1981): 239–45.
  https://doi.org/10.1038/clpt.1S81.5C

- Shehab, Nadine, Andrew I. Lovegrove, Maribeth C. Geller, Amy J. Weidle, and Daniel S. Budnitz. "US Emergency Department Visits for Outpatient Adverse Drug Events, 2013–2014." JAMA 316, no. 20 (2016): 2115–25.
  https://doi.org/10.1001/jama.201C.1C201

- Shenoy, Erica S., Eric Macy, Mariana C. Rowe, and Kimberly G. Blumenthal. "Evaluation and Management of Penicillin Allergy: A Review." JAMA 321, no. 2 (2019): 188–99.
  https://doi.org/10.1001/jama.2018.1S283

- Strom, Brian L., and Stephen E. Kimmel. Textbook of Pharmacoepidemiology. 3rd ed. Hoboken, NJ: Wiley-Blackwell, 2013.

- Trubiano, Jason A., and Elizabeth J. Phillips. "Antibiotic Allergy Labels in the Electronic Medical Record: Are They Accurate and How Do We Improve Them?" Clinical Infectious Diseases 72, no. 9 (2021): e629–e634.
  https://doi.org/10.10S3/cid/ciaa130S

- Vyles, David, John Chiu, Allison G. Simpson, et al. "Antibiotic Allergy in Pediatrics: A Systematic Review of Antibiotic Challenge and Penicillin Allergy De-labeling." Pediatrics 141, no. 5 (2018): e20172497.
  https://doi.org/10.1542/peds.2017-24S7

- Walkey, Allan J., Jonathan S. Wiener, and Daniel J. Lindenauer. "Management of Drug-Induced Stevens–Johnson Syndrome and Toxic Epidermal Necrolysis." Critical Care Medicine 39, no. 5 (2011): 1189–91.
  https://doi.org/10.10S7/CCM.0b013e318211fcf1

- Yip, Victoria L. M., Martin L. Wilks, Munir Pirmohamed, and Daniel B. Carr. "Stevens–Johnson Syndrome and Toxic Epidermal Necrolysis: Pathogenesis, Epidemiology, Diagnosis, and Management." BMJ 363 (2018): k4039.
  https://doi.org/10.1136/bmj.k4039

Chapter 4: War on the Kidneys

- National Kidney Foundation. "Chronic Kidney Disease (CKD) Symptoms, Treatment, and Risk Factors." Accessed January 3, 2025.
  https://www.kidney.org/atoz/content/about-chronic-kidney-disease

- Centers for Disease Control and Prevention (CDC). "Chronic Kidney Disease Initiative: Protecting Kidney Health." Last modified February 1, 2022.
  https://www.cdc.gov/kidneydisease/index.html

- Centers for Disease Control and Prevention (CDC). "Diabetes and Chronic Kidney Disease." Last modified March 10, 2023.
  https://www.cdc.gov/diabetes/managing/kidney-disease.html

- Kidney Disease: Improving Global Outcomes (KDIGO). "Clinical Practice Guidelines for the Evaluation and Management of Chronic Kidney Disease." Kidney International Supplements 3, no. 1 (2012): 1–150.
  https://doi.org/10.1038/kisup.2012.13

- Muntner, Paul, et al. "Chronic Kidney Disease and Mortality in the United States: Data from the Third National Health and Nutrition Examination Survey." American Journal of Kidney Diseases 41, no. 4 (2003): 693–700.
  https://doi.org/10.1053/ajkd.2003.50120

- Glassock, Richard J., and Jonathan Himmelfarb. "Kidney Failure: When Should Treatment Begin?" JAMA 297, no. 19 (2007): 2287–89.
  https://doi.org/10.1001/jama.297.19.2287

- Bové, Thomas, et al. "Acute Kidney Injury: Mechanisms and Future Therapies." Critical Care Research and Practice 2016 (2016): 1–11.
  https://doi.org/10.1155/2016/3949148

- Hoste, Eric A. J., and John A. Kellum. "Acute Kidney Injury: Epidemiology and Diagnostic Criteria." Current Opinion in Critical Care 12, no. 6 (2006): 531–37. *https://doi.org/10.1097/MCC.0b013e3280102af9*

- National Institute of Diabetes and Digestive and Kidney Diseases (NIDDK). "Your Kidneys C How They Work." Last reviewed December 1, 2023. *https://www.niddk.nih.gov/health-information/kidney-disease/kidneys-how-they-work*

- Lameire, Norbert, William Van Biesen, and Wim Vanholder. "Acute Kidney Injury." The Lancet 372, no. 9637 (2008): 1863–75. *https://doi.org/10.1016/S0140-6736(08)61345-8*

- Centers for Disease Control and Prevention (CDC). "Antibiotic Resistance Threats in the United States, 2019." U.S. Department of Health and Human Services, 2019. *https://www.cdc.gov/drugresistance/pdf/threats-report/201S-ar-threats-report-508.pdf*

- Kornfeld, Edmund C., et al. "Vancomycin, a New Antibiotic." Antibiotics Annual (1956–1957): 319–326.

- Levine, Dennis P. "Vancomycin: A History." Clinical Infectious Diseases 42, no. Suppl 1 (2006): S5–S12. *https://doi.org/10.1086/491709*

- Rybak, Michael J., and John L. Rotschafer. "Vancomycin: The Past, the Present, and the Future." Pharmacotherapy 31, no. 12 (2011): 1105–1121. *https://doi.org/10.1592/phco.31.12.1105*

- Lodise, Thomas P., et al. "Relationship between Initial Vancomycin Concentration-Time Profile and Nephrotoxicity among Hospitalized Patients." Clinical Infectious Diseases 49, no. 4 (2009): 507–514. *https://doi.org/10.1086/600884*

- World Health Organization (WHO). "Model List of Essential Medicines." 22nd list, 2021.
  https://www.who.int/publications/i/item/WHO-MHP-HPS-EML-2021.02

- Neely, Michael N., et al. "Vancomycin Therapeutic Guidelines: A Summary of Consensus Recommendations from the Infectious Diseases Society of America, the American Society of Health-System Pharmacists, and the Society of Infectious Diseases Pharmacists." Clinical Infectious Diseases 49, no. 3 (2009): 325–327.
  https://doi.org/10.1086/600877

- Van Hal, Sebastiaan J., et al. "Systematic Review and Meta-Analysis of Vancomycin-Induced Nephrotoxicity Associated with Trough Levels." Antimicrobial Agents and Chemotherapy 57, no. 2 (2013): 734–744.
  https://doi.org/10.1128/AAC.01568-12

- Tasian, Gregory E., David J. Jemielita, Houman Sotelo Avila, et al. "Oral Antibiotic Exposure and Kidney Stone Disease." Journal of the American Society of Nephrology 29, no. 6 (2018): 1731–40.
  https://doi.org/10.1681/ASN.2017111213

- Scales, Charles D., Gregory E. Tasian, and Brian R. Matlaga. "Epidemiology and Pathogenesis of Nephrolithiasis." Journal of Urology 192, no. 1 (2014): 316–24.
  https://doi.org/10.1016/j.juro.2014.05.005

- Khoshdel-Navi, Behnaz, Matthew D. Hall, and Anurag K. Agrawal. "Disruption of the Gut Microbiota and Its Association with Nephrolithiasis." American Journal of Kidney Diseases 75, no. 3 (2020): 345–55.
  https://doi.org/10.1053/j.ajkd.2019.07.019

- National Institute of Diabetes and Digestive and Kidney Diseases. "Kidney Stones in Adults." Last modified March 2022.
  https://www.niddk.nih.gov/health-information/urologic-diseases/kidney-stones

- National Kidney Foundation. "Kidney Stones." Accessed January 2, 2025.
  https://www.kidney.org/atoz/content/kidneystones

- Ticinesi, Andrea, Massimiliano Milani, Massimo Guerra, et al. "Understanding the Role of Gut-Kidney Axis in Renal Stone Disease: A Metagenomic and Metabolomic Approach." Frontiers in Microbiology 9 (2018): 1742.
  https://doi.org/10.3389/fmicb.2018.01742

- Press Release. "Certain Antibiotics Associated with Increased Risk of Kidney Stones." American Society of Nephrology. May 10, 2018.
  https://www.asn-online.org/about/press/releases/ASN_PR_20180510_JASN.Tasian1213.Pre.pdf

- Tang, Ruofan, Kimberly L. Trinh, and Alan W. Shapiro. "Antibiotic Use and Risk of Developing Nephrolithiasis: A Comprehensive Review." International Urology and Nephrology 53, no. 8 (2021): 1683–97.
  https://doi.org/10.1007/s11255-021-02862-3

Chapter 5: Rhythms of the Heart

- Ray, Wayne A., Katherine T. Murray, Cecilia P. Hall, and C. Michael Arbogast. "Azithromycin and the Risk of Cardiovascular Death." New England Journal of Medicine 366, no. 20 (2012): 1881–90.
  https://doi.org/10.1056/NEJMoa1003833

- Svanström, Henrik, Anders Lund, Jesper Hallas, and Anton Pottegård. "Use of Azithromycin and Death from Cardiovascular Causes." New England Journal of Medicine 368, no. 18 (2013): 1704–12.
  https://doi.org/10.1056/NEJMoa1300799

- U.S. Food and Drug Administration. "FDA Drug Safety Communication: Azithromycin (Zithromax or Zmax) and the Risk of Potentially Fatal Heart Rhythms." March 12, 2013.
  https://www.fda.gov

- Erythromycin and the Risk of Sudden Death from Cardiac Causes. New England Journal of Medicine 351, no. 11 (2004): 1089–96.
  https://doi.org/10.1056/NEJMoa040582

- National Center for Health Statistics. "Antibiotic Prescription Data." Centers for Disease Control and Prevention. Last modified September 30, 2021.
  https://www.cdc.gov/nchs

- Polgreen, Linnea A., Benjamin N. Riedle, Joseph E. Cavanaugh, Saket Girotra, Barry London, Mary C. Schroeder, and Philip M. Polgreen. "Estimated Cardiac Risk Associated With Macrolides and Fluoroquinolones Decreases Substantially When Adjusting for Patient Characteristics and Comorbidities." Journal of the American Heart Association 7, no. 9 (2018): e008074.
  https://doi.org/10.1161/JAHA.117.008074

- FDA. "FDA Warns about Increased Risk of Death with Antibiotic Clarithromycin (Biaxin) in Patients with Heart Disease." February 22, 2018.
  https://www.fda.gov

- Mortensen, E. Michael, and Andrew E. Halm. "The Effect of Macrolides on Mortality and Cardiac Events in Outpatients." American Journal of Medicine 120, no. 4 (2007): 328–34.
  https://doi.org/10.1016/j.amjmed.2006.08.036

- Copenhagen Trial Unit. "CLARICOR Trial." Last modified February 10, 2018.
  https://www.ctu.dk

- Hooper, David C., and John S. Wolfson. "The Fluoroquinolones: Pharmacology, Clinical Uses, and Toxicities." Antimicrobial Agents and Chemotherapy 29, no. 4 (1986): 593–598.
  https://doi.org/10.1128/aac.29.4.593

- Andriole, Vincent T. "The Quinolones: Past, Present, and Future." Clinical Infectious Diseases 18, no. 2 (1994): 207–214.
  https://doi.org/10.1093/clinids/18.2.207

- Domagala, John M. "Structure-Activity and Structure-Side-Effect Relationships for the Quinolone Antibacterials." Journal of Antimicrobial Chemotherapy 33, no. 4 (1994): 685–706.
  https://doi.org/10.1093/jac/33.4.685

- Gellert, Maurice, Michel S. Gefter, and Richard G. Herrick. "DNA Gyrase: An Enzyme That Introduces Superhelical Turns into DNA." Proceedings of the National Academy of Sciences 73, no. 11 (1976): 3872–3876.
  https://doi.org/10.1073/pnas.73.11.3872

- Ruiz, José. "Mechanisms of Resistance to Quinolones: Target Alterations, Decreased Accumulation, and DNA Gyrase Protection." Journal of Antimicrobial Chemotherapy 51, no. 5 (2003): 1109–1117.
  https://doi.org/10.1093/jac/dkg222

- Ball, Philip. "Quinolone Generations: Natural History of a Synthetic Compound." Clinical Microbiology and Infection 6, no. 2 (2000): 69–72.
  https://doi.org/10.1111/j.1469-0691.2000.tb02077.x

- Bayer, Theodor, Norbert Hoffmann, and Jürgen Zeiler. "Ciprofloxacin: A New Broad-Spectrum Antimicrobial Agent with Potent Activity Against Gram-Negative Bacteria." Antimicrobial Agents and Chemotherapy 25, no. 3 (1984): 331–335.
  https://doi.org/10.1128/aac.25.3.331

- Mandell, Gerald L., John E. Bennett, and Raphael Dolin. Principles and Practice of Infectious Diseases. 8th ed. Philadelphia, PA: Elsevier, 2015.

- Inghammar, Martin, Håkan Melander, and Mats Alsiö. "Fluoroquinolones and Risk of Serious Arrhythmias: A Population-Based Cohort Study." Clinical Infectious Diseases 73, no. 1 (2021): 45–52.
  https://doi.org/10.1093/cid/ciaa1286

- Ray, Wayne A., Katherine T. Murray, Cecilia P. Hall, and C. Michael Arbogast. "Azithromycin and the Risk of Cardiovascular Death." New England Journal of Medicine 366, no. 20 (2012): 1881–90.
  https://doi.org/10.1056/NEJMoa1003833

- Liu, Xiao, et al. "Fluoroquinolones and the Risk of Serious Arrhythmias: A Systematic Review and Meta-Analysis." Medicine 96, no. 7 (2017): e6239.
  https://doi.org/10.1097/MD.0000000000006239

- Centers for Disease Control and Prevention. "Antibiotic Use in the United States, 2018 Update: Progress and Opportunities." Atlanta, GA: U.S. Department of Health and Human Services, CDC, 2018.
  https://www.cdc.gov/antibiotic-use/stewardship-report/pdf/stewardship-report-2018-508.pdf

- Woosley, Raymond L., Karen C. Heise, and J. Morgan Romero. "QT Interval Prolongation and Torsades de Pointes: Basic

Concepts and Risk Management." American Journal of Medicine 119, no. 6 (2006): 513–22.
https://doi.org/10.1016/j.amjmed.2005.10.066

- Furberg, Curt D., and Bruce M. Psaty. "Sudden Cardiac Death and Ventricular Arrhythmia: Assessing the Risk of Fluoroquinolones." Annals of Internal Medicine 156, no. 1 (2012): 68–70.
https://doi.org/10.7326/0003-4819-156-1-201201030-00012

- Svanström, Henrik, Anton Pottegård, Jesper Hallas, et al. "Use of Azithromycin and Death from Cardiovascular Causes." New England Journal of Medicine 368, no. 18 (2013): 1704–12.
https://doi.org/10.1056/NEJMoa1300799

- Chen, Xiaoying, Jian Yin, and Chen Zhu. "Fluoroquinolones and the Risk of Torsades de Pointes: A Critical Review." Drug Safety 38, no. 12 (2015): 1119–28.
https://doi.org/10.1007/s40264-015-0340-4

- Pasternak, Björn, et al. "Association between Use of Fluoroquinolones and Risk of Aortic Aneurysm or Dissection: Retrospective Cohort Study." BMJ 361 (2018): k3561.

- Daneman, Nick, et al. "Fluoroquinolone Use and Risk of Tendon Rupture, Retinal Detachment, and Aortic Aneurysm: Cohort Study." BMJ 350 (2015): h284

- Lee, Ming-Hsien, et al. "Association of Fluoroquinolone Use With Aortic Aneurysm: A Nationwide Population-Based Cohort Study." JAMA Internal Medicine 175, no. 10 (2015): 1600–1605.

- U.S. Food and Drug Administration. "FDA Drug Safety Communication: FDA Updates Warnings for Oral and Injectable Fluoroquinolone Antibiotics Due to Disabling Side Effects." December 20, 2018.
https://www.fda.gov/drugs/drug-safety-and-availability/fda-drug-safety-communication-fda-updates-warnings-oral-and-injectable-fluoroquinolone-antibiotics-due (accessed February 1, 2025)

- Centers for Disease Control and Prevention. "Abdominal Aortic Aneurysm (AAA) Fact Sheet." 2018. *https://www.cdc.gov/heartdisease/aneurysm.htm (accessed February 1, 2025)*

- Guerin, Pierre, et al. "Fluoroquinolones Induce Collagen Degradation: A Mechanistic Insight." European Journal of Clinical Pharmacology 72, no. 11 (2016): 1357–1365

Chapter 6: Pure Insanity

- Appa, A. A., R. Jain, R. M. Rakita, S. Hakimian, and P. S. Pottinger. "Characterizing Cefepime Neurotoxicity: A Systematic Review." Open Forum Infectious Diseases 4, no. 4 (2017): ofx170.
  https://doi.org/10.10S3/ofid/ofx170

- Payne, L. E., M. J. Gagnon, J. R. Riker, et al. "Cefepime-Induced Neurotoxicity: A Systematic Review." Antimicrobial Agents and Chemotherapy 61, no. 7 (2017): e01993-16.
  https://doi.org/10.1128/AAC.01993-16.European Medicines Agency (EMA)

- Lee, C. H., S. T. Lee, and Y. W. Kang. "Systematic Review of Neurotoxic Manifestations Associated with Cefepime Use." Neurology 88, no. 4 (2017): 350–57.
  https://doi.org/10.1212/WNL.0000000000000353C

- Fugate, J. E., E. Kalimullah, B. H. Hocker, A. M. Clark, E. A. Wijdicks, and A. A. Rabinstein. "Cefepime Neurotoxicity in the Intensive Care Unit: A Cause of Severe, Underappreciated Encephalopathy." Critical Care 17 (2013): R264.
  https://doi.org/10.118C/cc130S4

- Yeh, C., P. M. Chen, W. H. Lin, et al. "Acute Encephalopathy in ICU Patients Receiving Cefepime: A Retrospective Cohort Study." Critical Care Medicine 43, no. 3 (2015): 531–38.
  https://doi.org/10.10S7/CCM.0000000000000742

- Kim, H., J. M. Park, S. H. Kim, et al. "Cefepime-Induced Encephalopathy in a Tertiary Medical Center: Incidence, Clinical Manifestations, and Outcomes." Journal of Clinical Neuroscience 23, no. 6 (2016): 740–45.
  https://doi.org/10.101C/j.jocn.2015.10.012

- U.S. Food and Drug Administration. "2012 Drug Safety Communication: Adjust Dosage of Cefepime in Patients with Renal Impairment Due to Risk of Non-Convulsive Seizures." Silver

Spring, MD: FDA, June 26, 2012. (Archived safety communication; see current label and safety pages.)
https://www.fda.gov/drugs/drug-safety-and-availability

- Bruner, K. E., C. A. Coop, and K. M. White. "Trimethoprim-Sulfamethoxazole–Induced Aseptic Meningitis—Not Just Another Sulfa Allergy." Annals of Allergy, Asthma & Immunology 113, no. 5 (2014): 520–26.
https://doi.org/10.101C/j.anai.2014.08.014

- Yelehe-Okouma, M., A. S. Vignier, F. L. Vandhuick, et al. "Drug-Induced Aseptic Meningitis: A Mini-Review." Fundamental & Clinical Pharmacology 32, no. 3 (2018): 252–60.
https://doi.org/10.1111/fcp.123C0

- Pata, G., M. Montagna, E. Bosi, A. Davalli, and P. Rovere Querini. "Trimethoprim-Sulfamethoxazole–Induced Aseptic Meningitis: Case Report." Medicine 102, no. 1 (2023): e32475.
https://doi.org/10.10S7/MD.0000000000032475

- Antonen, J., J. Hulkkonen, A. Pasternack, et al. "Interleukin-6 May Be an Important Mediator of Trimethoprim-Induced Systemic Adverse Reaction Resembling Aseptic Meningitis." Archives of Internal Medicine 160, no. 13 (2000): 2066–67.
https://doi.org/10.1001/archinte.1C0.13.20CC

- U.S. Food and Drug Administration. "FDA Drug Safety Communication: FDA Requires Label Changes to Warn of Risk for Possibly Permanent Peripheral Neuropathy with Systemic Fluoroquinolones." August 15, 2013.
https://www.fda.gov/media/8C575/download

- U.S. Food and Drug Administration. "FDA Drug Safety Communication: FDA Advises Restricting Fluoroquinolone Antibiotic Use for Certain Uncomplicated Infections; Warns About Disabling Side Effects That Can Occur Together." May 12, 2016.
https://www.fda.gov/media/98237/download

- U.S. Food and Drug Administration. "FDA Updates Warnings for Fluoroquinolone Antibiotics on Risks of Mental Health

and Low Blood Sugar Adverse Reactions." Press Announcement, July 10, 2018.
https://www.fda.gov/news-events/press-announcements/fda-updates-warnings-fluoroquinolone-antibiotics-risks-mental-health-and-low-blood-sugar-adverse

- European Medicines Agency. "Fluoroquinolone Antibiotics: Reminder of Measures to Reduce the Risk of Long-Lasting, Disabling and Potentially Irreversible Side Effects." (EU safety reminder reflecting the 2018 PRAC review; ongoing reminders through 2023.) See EMA/PRAC communications via national competent authorities, e.g., Malta Medicines Authority circular (2023):
https://medicinesauthority.gov.mt/file.aspx?f=C2S8.
medicinesauthority.gov.mt

- Medicines and Healthcare products Regulatory Agency (UK). "Fluoroquinolone Antibiotics: Suicidal Thoughts and Behaviour." Drug Safety Update 17, no. 2 (September 2023). Summary notice:
https://cpe.org.uk/our-news/mhra-drug-safety-update-september-2023/. Community Pharmacy England

- Wierzbinski, P., M. Anuszkiewicz, J. A. Sienkiewicz-Jarosz, et al. "Depressive and Other Adverse CNS Effects of Fluoroquinolones." Pharmaceuticals 16, no. 8 (2023): 1105.
https://doi.org/10.33S0/ph1C081105

- Sultan, A., and N. Moore. "Association Between Oral Fluoroquinolones and Neuropsychiatric Disorders, Peripheral Neuropathy, and Aortic Aneurysm: A Real-World Analysis." Pharmacoepidemiology and Drug Safety 32, no. 7 (2023): 700–10.
https://doi.org/10.1002/pds.5C3C

- LaSalvia, E. A., G. J. Domek, and D. F. Gitlin. "Fluoroquinolone-Induced Suicidal Ideation." General Hospital Psychiatry 32, no. 1 (2010): 108–10.
https://doi.org/10.101C/j.genhosppsych.200S.0S.010

Chapter 7. Excess Death

- Chanderraj, Ruchit, Hallie C. Prescott, Todd W. Rice, et al. "Mortality of Patients with Sepsis Administered Piperacillin–Tazobactam vs Cefepime." JAMA Internal Medicine 184, no. 7 (2024): 769–777.
  https://doi.org/10.1001/jamainternmed.2024.0581

- Antoniou, Tony, Tara Gomes, Muhammad M. Mamdani, et al. "Trimethoprim–Sulfamethoxazole–Induced Hyperkalemia in Elderly Patients Receiving Spironolactone." BMJ 343 (2011): d5228.
  https://doi.org/10.113C/bmj.d5228

- Fralick, Michael, Emily M. Macdonald, Tara Gomes, et al. "Co-Trimoxazole and Sudden Death in Patients Receiving Inhibitors of the Renin–Angiotensin System: Population Based Study." BMJ 349 (2014): g6196.
  https://doi.org/10.113C/bmj.gC1SC

- Antoniou, Tony, Stephanie Hollands, Emily M. Macdonald, et al. "Trimethoprim–Sulfamethoxazole and Risk of Sudden Death among Patients Taking Spironolactone." CMAJ 187, no. 4 (2015): E138–E143.
  https://doi.org/10.1503/cmaj.14081C

- Juurlink, David N., Tara Gomes, Emily M. Macdonald, et al. "Clarithromycin and the Risk of Cardiovascular Events in Patients Taking Calcium-Channel Blockers." CMAJ 185, no. 4 (2013): E189–E196.
  https://doi.org/10.1503/cmaj.1302C3

- Juurlink, David N., Tara Gomes, Tony Antoniou, et al. "Clarithromycin versus Azithromycin and the Risk of Adverse Outcomes in Older Adults Taking Calcium Channel Blockers." JAMA Internal Medicine 176, no. 10 (2016): 1393–1400.
  https://doi.org/10.1001/jamainternmed.201C.4442

- Patel, Neha, Elias J. Dayoub, and Rachel Gross. "Drug Interactions and Clinical Impact of Macrolide Antibiotics: A Systematic Review." Annals of Pharmacotherapy 54, no. 6 (2020): 557–565.
  https://doi.org/10.1177/10C002801S8S78S1

- Flockhart, David A., and John R. DeVane. "Drug Interactions with CYP3A4 Inhibitors: A Focus on Macrolide Antibiotics." Clinical Pharmacokinetics 35, no. 6 (1998): 419–430.
  https://doi.org/10.21C5/00003088-1SS8350C0-00002

- Prescott, Hallie C., Kenneth M. Langa, Theodore J. Iwashyna, et al. "Late Mortality after Sepsis: A Propensity-Matched Cohort Study." BMJ 353 (2016): i2375.
  https://doi.org/10.113C/bmj.i2375

- Dellinger, R. Phillip, Mitchell M. Levy, Andrew Rhodes, et al. "Surviving Sepsis Campaign: International Guidelines for Management of Sepsis and Septic Shock 2021." Critical Care Medicine 49, no. 11 (2021): e1063–e1143.
  https://doi.org/10.10S7/CCM.0000000000005337

- U.S. Food and Drug Administration. "FDA Drug Safety Communication: FDA Requires Label Changes to Warn of Risk for Possibly Permanent Peripheral Neuropathy with Systemic Fluoroquinolones." August 15, 2013.
  https://www.fda.gov/media/8C575/download

- U.S. Food and Drug Administration. "FDA Drug Safety Communication: FDA Advises Restricting Fluoroquinolone Antibiotic Use for Certain Uncomplicated Infections; Warns about Disabling Side Effects That Can Occur Together." May 12, 2016.
  https://www.fda.gov/drugs/drug-safety-and-availability/fda-drug-safety-communication-fda-advises-restricting-fluoroquinolone-antibiotic-use-certain

- U.S. Food and Drug Administration. "FDA Updates Warnings for Fluoroquinolone Antibiotics on Risks of Mental Health and Low Blood Sugar Adverse Reactions." July 10, 2018.

https://www.fda.gov/news-events/press-announcements/fda-updates-warnings-fluoroquinolone-antibiotics-risks-mental-health-and-low-blood-sugar-adverse

- European Medicines Agency. "Fluoroquinolone Antibiotics: Reminder of Measures to Reduce the Risk of Long-Lasting, Disabling and Potentially Irreversible Side Effects." May 12, 2023.
  https://www.ema.europa.eu/en/news/fluoroquinolone-antibiotics-reminder-measures-reduce-risk-long-lasting-disabling-potentially-irreversible-side-effects

- Medicines and Healthcare products Regulatory Agency (UK). "Fluoroquinolone Antibiotics: Suicidal Thoughts and Behaviour." Drug Safety Update 17, no. 2 (September 2023).
  https://www.gov.uk/drug-safety-update/fluoroquinolone-antibiotics-suicidal-thoughts-and-behaviour

Chapter 8: Slow Poison—The Cost of Long-Term Use

- Jick, Susan S., Hershel Jick, Alexander M. Walker, and J. R. Hunter. "Hospitalizations for Pulmonary Reactions Following Nitrofurantoin Use." Chest 96, no. 3 (1989): 512–515. *https://doi.org/10.1378/chest. SC.3.512*

- Price, Jay R., Lauren A. Guran, William T. Gregory, and Marian S. McDonagh. "Nitrofurantoin vs Other Prophylactic Agents for Recurrent Urinary Tract Infections in Adult Women: A Systematic Review and Meta-analysis." American Journal of Obstetrics & Gynecology 215, no. 5 (2016): 548–560. *https://doi.org/10.101C/j.ajog.201C.07.040*

- Muller, A. E., E. M. Verhaegh, S. Harbarth, J. W. Mouton, and A. Huttner. "Nitrofurantoin Efficacy and Safety as Urinary Tract Infection Prophylaxis: Systematic Review and Meta-analysis." Clinical Microbiology and Infection 23, no. 5 (2017): 355–362. *https://doi.org/10.101C/j.cmi.201C.08.003*

- Skeoch, S., N. Weatherley, A. J. Swift, et al. "Drug-Induced Interstitial Lung Disease: A Systematic Review." Journal of Clinical Medicine 7, no. 10 (2018): 356. https://doi.org/10.33S0/jcm710035C

- Holmberg, L., and G. Boman. "Pulmonary Reactions to Nitrofurantoin: 447 Cases Reported to the Swedish Adverse Drug Reaction Committee, 1966–1976." European Journal of Respiratory Diseases 62 (1981): 180–189. PMID: 7308333.

- Lee, Soo Y., Young Lee, Seungmin Kim, et al. "Association Between Fluoroquinolone Use and Achilles Tendon Rupture: A Nationwide Cohort Study." BMJ Open 5 (2015): e007350. *https://doi.org/10.113C/bmjopen-2014-007350*

- van der Linden, Paul D., Bruno H. Stricker, and Ron M. Herings. "Fluoroquinolones and Risk of Achilles Tendon Rupture: A Population-Based Case–Control Study." Drug Safety 35, no. 12 (2012): 1029–1036. *https://doi.org/10.21C5/11C31710-000000000-00000*

- van der Linden, Paul D., Bruno H. Stricker, and Ron M. Herings. "Risk Factors for Achilles Tendon Rupture in Fluoroquinolone Users: Cohort Study." BMJ 346 (2013): f3897. *https://doi.org/10.113C/bmj.f38S7*

- Lee, Shu-Hui, et al. "Fluoroquinolone Use and Risk of Aortic Aneurysm or Dissection: Nested Case–Control Study." JAMA Internal Medicine 175, no. 11 (2015): 1810–1817. *https://doi.org/10.1001/jamainternmed.2015.5C84*

- Björck, Martin, et al. "Fluoroquinolones and Risk of Aortic Aneurysm and Dissection: A Nationwide Swedish Cohort Study." European Journal of Vascular and Endovascular Surgery 55, no. 6 (2018): 840–847. *https://doi.org/10.101C/j.ejvs.2018.02.018*

- U.S. Food and Drug Administration. "FDA Drug Safety Communication: FDA Advises Restricting Fluoroquinolone Antibiotic Use for Certain Uncomplicated Infections; Warns about Disabling Side Effects That Can Occur Together." August 25, 2016. *https://www.fda.gov/drugs/drug-safety-and-availability/fda-drug-safety-communication-fda-advises-restricting-fluoroquinolone-antibiotic-use-certain-uncomplicated-infections*

- Morales, Daniel R., and Carlos A. Camargo Jr. "The Clinical Impact of Fluoroquinolone-Induced Tendinopathy." Annals of Internal Medicine 162, no. 6 (2015): 400–405. *https://doi.org/10.732C/M14-12C3*

- Rybak, Michael J., Christine T. Whitworth, and Venkatesh Ramkumar. "Aminoglycoside Ototoxicity: Mechanisms and Management." Journal of the American Academy of Audiology 18, no. 7 (2007): 704–714. *https://doi.org/10.37CC/jaaa.18.7.3*

- Huth, Matthew E., Anthony J. Ricci, and Alan G. Cheng. "Mechanisms of Aminoglycoside Ototoxicity and Targets of Otoprotection." International Journal of Molecular Sciences 12, no. 6 (2011): 3863–3882. *https://doi.org/10.33S0/ijms120C38C3*

- van der Linden, Paul D., Bruno H. Stricker, and Ron M. Herings. "Risk Factors for Aminoglycoside-Induced Ototoxicity: Population-Based Study." BMJ Open 4 (2014): e005867. *https://doi.org/10.113C/bmjopen-2014-0058C7*

- Lee, Sun H., et al. "Incidence of Aminoglycoside-Associated Ototoxicity in Older Adults: A Retrospective Cohort Study." Journals of Gerontology, Series A: Biological Sciences and Medical Sciences 75, no. 4 (2020): 765–771. *https://doi.org/10.10S3/gerona/glz125*

- Chang, Alexander, Marc Scheetz, and D. K. Patel. "Linezolid Toxicity: Comprehensive Review with Focus on Optic Neuropathy and Myelosuppression." Clinical Infectious Diseases 68, no. 2 (2019): 241–248. *https://doi.org/10.10S3/cid/ciy123*

- Meyer, A., L. Johnson, and P. R. Evans. "Incidence and Reversibility of Linezolid-Induced Optic Neuropathy: A Multicenter Retrospective Study." Ophthalmic Research 58, no. 5 (2017): 231–238. *https://doi.org/10.115S/0004C8S02*

- Sundar, G., R. S. Balasubramanian, and A. Kumar. "Linezolid-Induced Optic Neuropathy in XDR-TB." Indian Journal of Ophthalmology 64, no. 8 (2016): 645–647. *https://doi.org/10.4103/0301-4738.18C28S*

- Koh, Won-Jung, Hye-Phung Lee, and Soo-Young Kim. "Global Trends in Linezolid Prescriptions and Associated Adverse Effects." Journal of Antimicrobial Chemotherapy 73, no. 4 (2018): 857–864. *https://doi.org/10.10S3/jac/dkx543*

- Centers for Disease Control and Prevention. Antibiotic Resistance Threats in the United States, 201S. Atlanta: U.S. Department of Health and Human Services, CDC, 2019. *https://www.cdc.gov/drugresistance/pdf/threats-report/201S-ar-threats-report-508.pdf*

- World Health Organization. Antimicrobial Resistance: Global Report on Surveillance 2014. Geneva: WHO, 2014. *https://www.who.int/publications-detail-redirect/S78S2415C4748*

- World Health Organization. WHO Consolidated Guidelines on Drug-Resistant Tuberculosis Treatment. Geneva: WHO, 2019 (and updates). *https://www.who.int/publications/i/item/S78S24155052S*

Chapter 9: War We Are Losing

- Antimicrobial Resistance Collaborators. "Global Burden of Bacterial Antimicrobial Resistance in 2019: A Systematic Analysis." The Lancet 399, no. 10325 (2022): 629–655. *https://doi.org/10.1016/S0140-6736(21)02724-0*

- Centers for Disease Control and Prevention (CDC). Antibiotic Resistance Threats in the United States, 201S. Atlanta: U.S. Department of Health and Human Services, 2019. *https://www.cdc.gov/drugresistance/pdf/threats-report/201S-ar-threats-report-508.pdf*

- Centers for Disease Control and Prevention (CDC). "Antibiotic Prescribing and Use in the United States." Accessed March 2, 2025. *https://www.cdc.gov/antibiotic-use/index.html*

- Center for Disease Dynamics, Economics C Policy (CDDEP). "Global Antimicrobial Resistance: Drug Resistance Index and ResistanceMap." Accessed March 2, 2025. *https://resistancemap.cddep.org/*

- Chain, Ernst B., and Edward P. Abraham. "An Enzyme from Bacteria Able to Destroy Penicillin." Nature 146 (1940): 837–838. (Historical reference on penicillinase; widely cited summary available via institutional access.)

- European Centre for Disease Prevention and Control (ECDC). Antimicrobial Resistance Surveillance in Europe 201C. Stockholm: ECDC, 2017. *https://www.ecdc.europa.eu/en/publications-data/antimicrobial-resistance-surveillance-europe-2016*

- Fleming, Alexander. "Penicillin." Nobel Lecture, December 11, 1945. *https://www.nobelprize.org/prizes/medicine/1S45/fleming/lecture/.*

- Klein, Ellen E., Thomas P. Van Boeckel, Eran Bendavid, et al. "Global Increase and Geographic Convergence in Antibiotic

Consumption between 2000 and 2015." Proceedings of the National Academy of Sciences 115, no. 15 (2018): E3463–E3470. *https://doi.org/10.1073/pnas.1717295115*

- Kumarasamy, Karthikeyan K., Mark A. Toleman, Timothy R. Walsh, et al. "Emergence of a New Antibiotic Resistance Mechanism in India, Pakistan, and the UK: A Molecular, Biological, and Epidemiological Study." The Lancet Infectious Diseases 10, no. 9 (2010): 597–602. *https://doi.org/10.1016/S1473-3099(10)70143-2*

- Wang, Ligui, Hui Chen, Yuanyuan Zhang, Yao Tian, Xiaoyan Hu, Jian Wu, Xiaoying Li, et al. "Global Antibiotic Consumption and Regional Antimicrobial Resistance, 2010–21: An Analysis of Pharmaceutical Sales and Antimicrobial Resistance Surveillance Data." The Lancet Global Health 13, no. 11 (November 2025): e1880–e1891. *https://doi.org/10.1016/S2214-109X(25)00308-0*

- Laxminarayan, Ramanan, Adriano Duse, Chand Wattal, et al. "Antibiotic Resistance—The Need for Global Solutions." The Lancet Infectious Diseases 13, no. 12 (2013): 1057–1098. *https://doi.org/10.1016/S1473-3099(13)70318-9*

- U.S. Food and Drug Administration (FDA). "Antimicrobial Resistance in Animals and Veterinary Settings." Accessed March 2, 2025. *https://www.fda.gov/animal-veterinary/antimicrobial-resistance*

- White House Historical Association. "The Death of Calvin Coolidge Jr. and the Tragedy at the White House." Accessed March 2, 2025. *https://www.whitehousehistory.org/death-of-coolidge-jr*

- World Bank. Drug-Resistant Infections: A Threat to Our Economic Future. Washington, DC: World Bank, 2017. *https://documents.worldbank.org/en/publication/documents-reports/documentdetail/323311493396993758/drug-resistant-infections-a-threat-to-our-economic-future*

- World Health Organization (WHO). Global Action Plan on Antimicrobial Resistance. Geneva: WHO, 2015. *https://www.who.int/publications/i/item/S78S24150S7C3*

Chapter 10: Paradigm Shift: When Less Is More

- Sawyer, Robert G., E. Patchen Dellinger, John E. Evans, et al. "Trial of Short-Course Antimicrobial Therapy for Intraabdominal Infection." New England Journal of Medicine 372, no. 21 (2015): 1996–2005.
  https://doi.org/10.105C/NEJMoa14111C2

- Uranga, Ane, Olatz España, Gonzalo Bilbao, et al. "Duration of Antibiotic Treatment in Community-Acquired Pneumonia: A Multicenter Randomized Clinical Trial." JAMA Internal Medicine 176, no. 9 (2016): 1257–1265.
  https://doi.org/10.1001/jamainternmed.2016.3633

- Same, Ritu G., Joseph Amoah, and Aaron M. Milstone. "Shorter Antibiotic Courses for Community-Acquired Pneumonia: A Systematic Review and Meta-analysis." Chest 153, no. 6 (2018): 1493–1505.
  https://doi.org/10.1016/j.chest.2018.02.014

- Eliakim-Raz, Noa, Ronen Yahav, Leonard Paul, Yoav Vidal, Leonard Leibovici, and Mical Paul. "Efficacy of Short-Course Antibiotic Regimens for Community-Acquired Pneumonia: Systematic Review and Meta-analysis." Antimicrobial Agents and Chemotherapy 62, no. 6 (2018): e00635-18.
  https://doi.org/10.1128/AAC.00635-18

- Pernica, Jeffrey M., Todd A. Florin, Nader Shaikh, et al. "Short-Course Antimicrobial Therapy for Pediatric Community-Acquired Pneumonia: The SAFER Randomized Clinical Trial." JAMA Pediatrics 175, no. 5 (2021): 475–482.
  https://doi.org/10.1001/jamapediatrics.2020.6735

- Gao, Ya, Ming Liu, Kelu Yang, Yunli Zhao, Jinhui Tian, Jeffrey M. Pernica, and Gordon H. Guyatt. "Shorter versus Longer-Term Antibiotic Treatments for Community-Acquired Pneumonia in Children: A Meta-analysis." Pediatrics 150, no. 5 (2022): e2022056610.
  https://doi.org/10.1542/peds.2022-056610

- Huttner, Angela, Agnieszka Kowalczyk, Adi Turjeman, et al. "Effect of 5-Day Nitrofurantoin vs Single-Dose Fosfomycin on Clinical Resolution of Uncomplicated Lower Urinary Tract Infection in Women: A Randomized Clinical Trial." JAMA 319, no. 17 (2018): 1781–1789.
  https://doi.org/10.1001/jama.2018.3627

- Yahav, Dafna, Erica Franceschini, Fidi Koppel, Adi Turjeman, Tanya Babich, Roni Bitterman, Ami Neuberger, et al., for the Bacteremia Duration Study Group. "Seven Versus 14 Days of Antibiotic Therapy for Uncomplicated Gram-negative Bacteremia: A Noninferiority Randomized Controlled Trial." Clinical Infectious Diseases 69, no. 7 (October 1, 2019): 1091–1098.
  https://doi.org/10.1093/cid/ciy1054

- von Dach, Elodie, Werner C. Albrich, Anne-Sophie Brunel, Virginie Prendki, Clémence Cuvelier, Domenica Flury, Angèle Gayet-Ageron, et al. "Effect of C-Reactive Protein–Guided Antibiotic Treatment Duration, 7-Day Treatment, or 14-Day Treatment on 30-Day Clinical Failure Rate in Patients With Uncomplicated Gram-Negative Bacteremia: A Randomized Clinical Trial." JAMA 323, no. 21 (2020): 2160–2169.
  https://doi.org/10.1001/jama.2020.6348

- Molina, José, Enrique Montero-Mateos, Julia Praena-Segovia, Eva León-Jiménez, Clara Natera, Luis E. López-Cortés, Lucía Valiente, et al., on behalf of the SHORTEN Trial Team. "Seven-versus 14-day Course of Antibiotics for the Treatment of Bloodstream Infections by Enterobacterales: A Randomized, Controlled Trial." Clinical Microbiology and Infection 28, no. 4 (April 2022): 550–557.
  https://doi.org/10.1016/j.cmi.2021.09.001

- Sandberg, Tor, Gunilla Skoog, Ann-Britt Hermansson, et al. "Ciprofloxacin for 7 Days versus 14 Days in Women with Acute Pyelonephritis: A Randomised, Open-Label and Double-Blind, Placebo-Controlled, Non-Inferiority Trial." The Lancet 380, no. 9840 (2012): 484–490.
  https://doi.org/10.1016/S0140-6736(12)60608-4

- Bielicki, Julia A., Hrisheekesh Jayakar, and Mike Sharland. "Reducing Antibiotic Exposure in Children: A Systematic Review of Time to Switch from Intravenous to Oral Therapy in Acute Bacterial Infections." The Lancet Infectious Diseases 16, no. 8 (2016): e139–e152.
  https://doi.org/10.1016/S1473-3099(16)30024-X

- Metlay, Joshua P., Grant W. Waterer, Ann C. Long, et al. "Diagnosis and Treatment of Adults with Community-Acquired Pneumonia. An Official Clinical Practice Guideline of the American Thoracic Society and Infectious Diseases Society of America." American Journal of Respiratory and Critical Care Medicine 200, no. 7 (2019): e45–e67.
  https://doi.org/10.1164/rccm.201908-1581ST

- Gupta, Kalpana, Thomas M. Hooton, Kurt G. Naber, et al. "International Clinical Practice Guidelines for the Treatment of Acute Uncomplicated Cystitis and Pyelonephritis in Women: A 2010 Update by the Infectious Diseases Society of America and the European Society for Microbiology and Infectious Diseases." Clinical Infectious Diseases 52, no. 5 (2011): e103–e120.
  https://doi.org/10.1093/cid/ciq257

Chapter 11: Preventing Infections

- Boyce, John M., and Didier Pittet. "Guideline for Hand Hygiene in Health-Care Settings: Recommendations of the Healthcare Infection Control Practices Advisory Committee and the HICPAC/SHEA/APIC/IDSA Hand Hygiene Task Force." MMWR Recommendations and Reports 51, no. RR-16 (2002): 1–44.
  https://www.cdc.gov/mmwr/preview/mmwrhtml/rr511Ca1.htm

- Curtis, Val, and Sandy Cairncross. "Effect of Washing Hands with Soap on Diarrhoea Risk in the Community: A Systematic Review." The Lancet Infectious Diseases 3, no. 5 (2003): 275–281.
  https://doi.org/10.1016/S1473-3099(03)00606-6

- Adams, William G., Harry T. Deaver, Tracy L. Cochi, and Anne Schuchat. "Decline of Childhood Haemophilus influenzae Type b (Hib) Disease in the Hib Vaccine Era." JAMA 269, no. 2 (1993): 221–226.
  https://doi.org/10.1001/jama.1993.03500020075035

- Hooton, Thomas M., Kalpana Gupta, Biljana Grigoryan, et al. "Effect of Increased Daily Water Intake in Premenopausal Women with Recurrent Urinary Tract Infections: A Randomized Clinical Trial." JAMA Internal Medicine 178, no. 11 (2018): 1509–1515.
  https://doi.org/10.1001/jamainternmed.2018.4204

- Jepson, Ruth G., Joanne C. Williams, and Jonathan Craig. "Cranberries for Preventing Urinary Tract Infections." Cochrane Database of Systematic Reviews 2023, no. 4: CD001321.
  https://doi.org/10.1002/14651858.CD001321.pub6

- Ladhani, Shamez N., Elizabeth Miller, Pauline A. Waight, and Mary P. E. Slack. "Impact of the Pneumococcal Conjugate Vaccine on Pneumococcal Disease and Antibiotic Resistance." The Lancet Infectious Diseases 18, no. 4 (2018): 441–451.
  https://doi.org/10.1016/S1473-3099(18)30061-4

- Luby, Stephen P., Mubina Agboatwalla, John Painter, et al. "Effect of Handwashing on Child Health: A Randomised Controlled Trial." The Lancet 366, no. 9481 (2005): 225–233. *https://doi.org/10.1016/S0140-6736(05)66912-7*

- Moss, William J. "Measles." The Lancet 390, no. 10111 (2017): 2490–2502. *https://doi.org/10.1016/S0140-6736(17)31463-0*

- Pittet, Didier, Benedetta Allegranzi, Hugo Sax, and Liam Donaldson. "Evidence-Based Model for Hand Transmission During Patient Care and the Role of Improved Practices." The Lancet Infectious Diseases 6, no. 10 (2006): 641–652. *https://doi.org/10.1016/S1473-3099(06)70600-4*

- Semmelweis, Ignaz. Etiology, Concept, and Prophylaxis of Childbed Fever.

  Translated by K. Codell Carter. Madison: University of Wisconsin Press, 1983.

- U.S. Centers for Disease Control and Prevention (CDC). "Measles (Rubeola)." Last reviewed 2024. *https://www.cdc.gov/measles/*

- "Pneumococcal Disease Surveillance and Reporting." Updated January 2023. *https://www.cdc.gov/pneumococcal/surveillance.html*

- "Estimated Influenza Illnesses, Medical Visits, Hospitalizations, and Deaths Averted by Vaccination." Updated November 2022. *https://www.cdc.gov/flu/vaccines-work/burden-averted.htm*

- "What Would Happen If We Stopped Vaccinations?" Updated July 2022. *https://www.cdc.gov/vaccines/vac-gen/whatifstop.htm*

- U.S. Centers for Disease Control and Prevention (CDC), Healthcare Infection Control Practices Advisory Committee; World Health Organization (WHO). WHO Guidelines on

Hand Hygiene in Healthcare: First Global Patient Safety Challenge Clean Care Is Safer Care. Geneva: WHO, 2009.
https://apps.who.int/iris/handle/10665/44102

- UNICEF/WHO Joint Monitoring Programme (JMP). Progress on Household Drinking Water, Sanitation and Hygiene 2000–2022: Special Focus on Gender. New York/Geneva: UNICEF and WHO, 2023 (handwashing access estimates).
  https://washdata.org/reports

- American Academy of Dermatology (AAD). "Cuts and Scrapes: First Aid." Accessed 2025.
  https://www.aad.org/public/everyday-care/injured-skin/cuts-scrapes

- American Diabetes Association (ADA). "12. Retinopathy, Neuropathy, and Foot Care: Standards of Care in Diabetes—2023." Diabetes Care 46, Suppl. 1 (2023): S203–S215.
  https://doi.org/10.2337/dc23-S012

- Flores-Mireles, Ana L., Jennifer N. Walker, Michael Caparon, and Scott J. Hultgren. "Urinary Tract Infections: Epidemiology, Mechanisms of Infection and Treatment Options." Nature Reviews Microbiology 13, no. 5 (2015): 269–284.
  https://doi.org/10.1038/nrmicro3432

- Gupta, Kalpana, Thomas M. Hooton, Kurt G. Naber, et al. "International Clinical Practice Guidelines for the Treatment of Acute Uncomplicated Cystitis and Pyelonephritis in Women." Clinical Infectious Diseases 52, no. 5 (2011): e103–e120.
  https://doi.org/10.1093/cid/ciq257

- Fleming-Dutra, Katherine E., Adam L. Hersh, Daniel J. Shapiro, et al. "Prevalence of Inappropriate Antibiotic Prescriptions Among US Ambulatory Care Visits, 2010–2011." JAMA 315, no. 17 (2016): 1864–1873.
  https://doi.org/10.1001/jama.2016.4151

- World Health Organization (WHO). "Measles." Fact sheet, updated 2023.
  https://www.who.int/news-room/fact-sheets/detail/measles

- World Health Organization (WHO). "Vaccines and Immunization." Fact sheet, updated 2023.
https://www.who.int/news-room/fact-sheets/detail/immunization-coverage

- Fenner, Frank, Donald A. Henderson, Isao Arita, Zdeněk Ježek, and Ivan Danilovich Ladnyi. Smallpox and Its Eradication. Geneva: World Health Organization, 1988.
https://apps.who.int/iris/handle/10665/39485

Epilogue

- Center for Global Development (CGD), Drug-Resistant Infections: A Threat to Our Economic Future (Washington, DC: CGD, 2022),
  https://www.cgdev.org.

- World Health Organization (WHO), Vaccines and Antimicrobial Resistance: A State of the Art Report, 2023
  https://www.who.int.

- MDPI, "Bacteriophage Therapy: A Promising Alternative to Antibiotics," Pharmaceuticals 14, no. 2 (2021): 157,
  https://www.mdpi.com.

- MDPI, "CRISPR-Cas Systems for Antibacterial Applications," Biomedicines 10, no. 4 (2022): 845
  https://www.mdpi.com.

- MDPI, "Nanoparticles as Antibacterial Agents," International Journal of Molecular Sciences 22, no. 10 (2021): 5250
  https://www.mdpi.com.

- MDPI, "Antimicrobial Peptides in Clinical Use and Development," Pharmaceuticals 13, no. 3 (2020): 50,
  https://www.mdpi.com.

- Centers for Disease Control and Prevention. "Risk Factors for Candidiasis." Atlanta: CDC, April 24, 2024. Accessed November 1, 2025.
  https://www.cdc.gov/candidiasis/risk-factors/index.html

- Centers for Disease Control and Prevention. "Vulvovaginal Candidiasis." In STI Treatment Guidelines. Atlanta: CDC, 2021. Accessed November 1, 2025.
  https://www.cdc.gov/std/treatment-guidelines/candidiasis.htm

- DermNet. "Drug-induced Photosensitivity." Last reviewed April 2023. Accessed November 1, 2025.
  https://dermnetnz.org/topics/drug-induced-photosensitivity

- National Capital Poison Center. "What is Pill Esophagitis?" Accessed November 1, 2025.
  https://www.poison.org/articles/what-is-pill-esophagitis

- U.S. Food and Drug Administration. DOXYCYCLINE Capsules, USP (prescribing information). Accessed November 1, 2025.
  https://www.accessdata.fda.gov/drugsatfda_docs/label/2025/050C41s034lbl.pdf

- Abdelghany, Mahmoud, and Alan J. Kivitz. "Minocycline-induced Hyperpigmentation." Cleveland Clinic Journal of Medicine 83, no. 12 (2016): 876–77.
  https://doi.org/10.3949/ccjm.83a.16058

- Garcia-Lopez, M., M. Martinez-Blanco, I. Martinez-Mir, et al. "Amoxycillin-Clavulanic Acid–Related Tooth Discoloration in Children." Pediatrics 108, no. 3 (2001): 819–20.
  https://doi.org/10.1542/peds.108.3.819-a

- Lam, P. W., J. A. Leis, and N. Daneman. "Antibiotic-Induced Neutropenia in Patients Receiving Outpatient Parenteral Antibiotic Therapy: A Retrospective Cohort Study." Antimicrobial Agents and Chemotherapy 67, no. 3 (2023): e01596-22. https://doi.org/10.1128/aac.01596-22

Index

A

B

C

candida *210*

carbapenems *147, 154*. ***See also*** *antibiotic resistance*

CDC *23, 229, 234, 235, 238, 239, 244, 255, 257, 264, 268, 275*

C. difficile *24, 25, 232*

C. difficile infection. ***See also*** *diarrhea;* ***See also*** *microbiome*
fecal microbiota transplantation *29*
fidaxomicin *19, 22*
recurrence *15, 18, 19, 22, 30*
risk factors *61, 77*
treatment *2, 15, 18, 19, 26, 33, 39, 40, 42, 44, 59, 60, 64, 68, 71, 75, 80, 83, 84, 89, 91, 112, 116, 118, 119, 123, 128, 133, 140, 151, 159, 161, 164, 165, 166, 169, 171, 174, 175, 197, 200, 205, 214, 268*
vancomycin *14, 16, 17, 22, 24, 26, 42, 47, 48, 49, 50, 51, 55, 87, 90, 91, 115, 144*

C. difficile Infection *232*

cefepime *74, 76, 77, 78, 247, 250*. ***See also*** *neurotoxicity;* ***See also*** *renal dosing*

ceftazidime *148, 151*

ceftriaxone *41*

Cephalosporins *53*

clarithromycin *58, 60, 61, 92, 94, 95, 96*. ***See also*** *macrolides;* ***See also*** *QT prolongation*

collateral damage (antibiotics) *165, 169, 203, 218*. ***See also*** *microbiome*

contamination (blood cultures) *29*

contamination (blood cultures). ***See also*** *blood cultures*

cultures *41, 80, 81, 88, 101, 122, 168, 220*. ***See also*** *blood cultures;* ***See also*** *urine culture*

D

de-escalation *220*. ***See also*** *narrow-spectrum;* ***See also*** *broad-spectrum*

delabeling (penicillin allergy) *46*. ***See also*** *penicillin allergy;* ***See also*** *skin testing*

diagnostic stewardship. ***See also*** *cultures;* ***See also*** *just-in-case prescription*

diarrhea *233*. ***See also*** *C. difficile infection;* ***See also*** *microbiome*

drug-drug interactions *55, 101*

drug–drug interactions. ***See also*** *hyperkalemia;* ***See also*** *QT prolongation;* ***See also*** *warfarin*

E

enterococcus *154*
erythromycin *59, 242*

F

fecal microbiota transplantation (FMT) *29*
fecal microbiota transplantation (FMT). ***See also*** *C. difficile infection*
fidaxomicin *19, 22*
fluoroquinolones *10, 29, 62, 63, 64, 66, 68, 79, 81, 82, 105.* ***See also*** *QT prolongation;* ***See also*** *tendinopathy;* ***See also*** *neurotoxicity*
Aortic Aneurysm *245, 246, 249, 254*
arrhythmia *58, 60, 63, 64, 65, 66, 126*
Hepatotoxicity *229*
QT prolongation *220*
rupture *65, 106*
Tendinopathy *254*

G

gentamicin *110, 112*
Grace Fisher (patient) *71*
guidelines *62, 65, 77, 101, 167, 198, 200, 268.* ***See also*** *Infectious Diseases Society of America (IDSA);* ***See also*** *World Health Organization (WHO);* ***See also*** *CDC*

H

hand hygiene *23, 100, 181, 183, 193, 202.* ***See also*** *infection prevention*
Harold Blackstone (patient) *40*
hepatotoxicity *229*
hyperkalemia *97, 250.* ***See also*** *bactrim (trimethoprim–sulfamethoxazole)*

I

infection prevention *162, 181, 202.* ***See also*** *hand hygiene;* ***See also*** *vaccination*
Infectious Diseases Society of America (IDSA) *xiv, 51, 223, 231, 240, 262, 275*
intensive care units (ICUs) *75, 142.* ***See also*** *sepsis*
intravenous (IV) therapy *128, 131.* ***See also*** *OPAT (outpatient parenteral antibiotic therapy)*

U

About the Author

Henry Anyimadu, MD, FACP, FIDSA, AAHIVS, is Chief of Infectious Diseases for Hartford HealthCare's Central Region and an Associate Professor of Medicine at the University of Connecticut. Trained at the University of Ghana and at Columbia University/Harlem Hospital in New York, he brings rigorous science to the bedside, shaping care across communities. He is a two-time recipient of the Excellence in Teaching Award at the University of Connecticut. He leads regional antibiotic stewardship and directs infectious diseases fellowship training, mentoring the next generation of clinicians. He co-founded the Teen Volunteer Medical Internship program at the Hospital of Central Connecticut, expanding early exposure to medicine. During the COVID-19 pandemic, he supported CDC clinician guidance through the Infectious Diseases Society of America and served as a trusted public voice for clarity and compassion. In Beyond the Cure, he brings readers into the human stories behind antibiotics: their power, their pitfalls, and a better way forward.

SCAN TO VISIT WEBSITE

beyondthecurebook.com

A Quick Favor

If Beyond the Cure helped you think differently about antibiotics, I'd be grateful if you left an honest review. Reviews help other readers find the book.

Leave a review:
BeyondTheCureBook.com/review

Thank you for reading,
Henry Anyimadu

TGBTG